Promoting Healthy Outcomes During Pregnancy and Beyond

This book provides essential knowledge and tools for home visitors and other parent-facing professionals to build trusting relationships with pregnant and postpartum clients, in order to provide them with the information, guidance, resources, and signposting they need to avoid adverse health outcomes. Adverse health outcomes as a result of pregnancy and birth affect millions each year, affecting physical and mental health – and in some cases resulting in death. Due to systemic bias and persistent socioeconomic disparities, certain groups are more at risk for these poor outcomes, including people of color, especially Black people; people from lower socioeconomic backgrounds; lesbian, gay, bisexual, transgender, and queer (LGBTQ+) people; and disabled people.

Sitting within a social determinants of health framework, this practical guide summarizes the most relevant research and translates it into action steps. Each chapter will address a key issue related to morbidity and mortality in relation to pregnancy and birth, including statistics, key definitions, and discussion of risk factors, protective factors, and disparities. Case studies, reflective questions, and recommendations make it straightforward for the reader to apply the learning to their own practice.

This book is an invaluable resource for all those health, community, and social service providers, including home visitors, who work with families, parents to be, and new parents.

Christina F. Mondi, PhD, is Instructor of Psychology at Harvard Medical School, USA; Lead Researcher and Evaluator at the Brazelton Touchpoints Center, Division of Developmental Medicine, Boston Children's Hospital, USA; and Affiliate Faculty in Global Health at Boston Children's Hospital, USA. She is a licensed psychologist and a preschool mental health consultant. Across domains, her work focuses on community – and school-based initiatives that support the mental health and well-being of young children and families.

Joanne Roberts, PhD, MBA, is Co-Director of Research and Evaluation at the Brazelton Touchpoints Center, Division of Developmental Medicine, Boston Children's Hospital, USA. She has over 20 years of experience in the field of early education and care, including research and consultative expertise related to both practice and policy. She has particular expertise in program quality evaluation and has worked extensively across diverse early childhood education programs, including community-based center care and family childcare.

Lindsey Sagasta, M.S.ED, MPH, is Child and Youth Violence Prevention Epidemiologist at the Massachusetts Department of Public Health, USA. Her background includes experience in early childhood education and as a research and evaluation coordinator at the Brazelton Touchpoints Center. Drawing on her extensive experience supporting initiatives in childhood development, violence prevention, and maternal morbidity and mortality, she aims to transform data into public health strategies that empower children, families, and communities to thrive.

Lindsay Boyer, MS, is Research Coordinator at the Brazelton Touchpoints Center, Division of Developmental Medicine, Boston Children's Hospital, USA. She began her career as a pre-kindergarten teacher and has since dedicated her time to supporting children and families outside of the classroom. Her experience includes providing technical assistance and evaluation services to family-facing providers, ranging from home visitors to early childhood educators.

Jillian Brashear, MPH, is Research Coordinator at the Brazelton Touchpoints Center, Division of Developmental Medicine, Boston Children's Hospital, USA. In this role, she supports community-based research projects focused on improving health outcomes and program quality from the perinatal period through early childhood. With a background in epidemiology and maternal and child health, she is passionate about the intersection of data and storytelling to address the social determinants of health affecting families and communities.

Allison Kemner, MPH, is Chief Research Officer and Senior Vice President at the Parents as Teachers National Center, USA. She directs the Parents as Teachers Research Council and collaborates with a network of researchers and university partners to conduct research, evaluation, and learning on the Parents as Teachers evidence-based home visiting model. She oversees data collection, analysis, and dissemination; guiding quality assurance, continuous improvement, and model innovation.

Sondra Horowitz, MA, is Senior Director of Quality Improvement at the Parents as Teachers National Center, USA. In this role, she oversees the organization's Quality Endorsement and Improvement Process and works on a variety of initiatives dedicated to translating home visiting research into practice.

Lindsey Shah, MSW, LCSW, is the Director of Content and Curricula at Parents as Teachers National Center. Her work focuses on providing high-quality, research-based information, strategies, and tools to support family engagement and home visiting professionals across the county. She is the lead author on Parents as Teachers publication *Engaged: Building Intentional Partnerships with Families.* Her previous experiences include roles that focus on mental health, both in education and pediatric emergency room settings.

Abigail Edwards, MPH, currently serves as Research and Data Specialist II at Parents as Teachers National Center, USA. In this role, she helps guide the organization's research and learning initiatives, including a project integrating doula services within the evidence-based home visiting model.

Kerry Caverly, BS, is Senior Vice President and Chief Program Officer at the Parents as Teachers National Center, USA. She oversees the coordination, integration, and delivery of all programs, contracts and related services, promoting collaborative relationships between Parents as Teachers National Center program areas. She also oversees the expansion and model replication and training, curriculum, and program development departments of Parents as Teachers.

Catherine Ayoub, EdD, MN, is Associate Professor at Harvard Medical School; Co-Director of Research and Evaluation and Director of Mental Health Consultation Services at the Brazelton Touchpoints Center, Division of Developmental Medicine, Boston Children's Hospital, USA. She is a licensed psychologist and nurse practitioner with 40 years of experience and 180 publications. Her primary interest is introducing and evaluating practice innovations to improve the care and life course of young children and families.

Promoting Healthy Outcomes During Pregnancy and Beyond

The Role of Community and Social Service Providers

Christina F. Mondi, Joanne Roberts, Lindsey Sagasta, Lindsay Boyer, Jillian Brashear, Allison Kemner, Sondra Horowitz, Lindsey Shah, Abigail Edwards, Kerry Caverly, and Catherine Ayoub

Routledge
Taylor & Francis Group
LONDON AND NEW YORK

Designed cover image: Amanda Million

First published 2026
by Routledge
4 Park Square, Milton Park, Abingdon, Oxon OX14 4RN

and by Routledge
605 Third Avenue, New York, NY 10158

Routledge is an imprint of the Taylor & Francis Group, an informa business

British Library Cataloguing-in-Publication Data
A catalogue record for this book is available from the British Library

ISBN: 978-1-032-75983-8 (hbk)
ISBN: 978-1-032-75968-5 (pbk)
ISBN: 978-1-003-47647-4 (ebk)

DOI: 10.4324/9781003476474

Typeset in Galliard
by Apex CoVantage, LLC

A mother's death is a searing, unimaginable tragedy, the effects of which last for decades . . . If we can turn the pain of maternal death into righteous indignation about the loss of something so precious, we can take action to ensure that for [future generations] . . . every birth is sacred and safe.

– Katy B. Kozhimannil (2018), "Reversing the Rise in Maternal Mortality".

This book is dedicated to the families who generously entrusted their stories to us and to all those who have experienced health complications or lost loved ones during pregnancy, childbirth, the postpartum period, or the first year of life. Our fervent hope is that this book will lift up your experiences and inspire increased supports for pregnant and postpartum individuals, babies, and their families moving forward.

Contents

Preface

The journey of pregnancy, childbirth, and early parenting is meant to be a time of hope and joy. Yet, for too many families around the world, it can become a time of uncertainty and fear. Too many mothers face serious health complications during pregnancy and after childbirth, complications that sometimes put their lives – and the lives of their babies – at risk. These challenges do not just affect individual families – they affect our communities and all of us.

Parents as Teachers (PAT) is an evidence-based early childhood education program designed to support families in their role as their child's first and most influential teachers. Founded in 1984, PAT provides parents with the resources, knowledge, and skills necessary to foster their children's healthy development and learning from birth through age 5. The program operates on the belief that parents are the most significant influence in their child's life, and through empowering them, families can build strong foundations for lifelong learning. PAT is one of many home visiting models that provide support to families during the prenatal and postpartum periods.

As the president and chief executive officer at PAT National Center, I have both a professional and personal connection to this topic. Professionally, PAT has been in the work of supporting birthing families since its inception. In 2014, we brought this work closest to the National Center by supporting our own affiliate, Show Me Strong Families – a lab school of sorts, to help keep us grounded in the intimate, everyday work with families, the management of an affiliate, and operationalizing implementation standards. In our own community in St. Louis, we know there is a public health crisis when it comes to morbidity and mortality before, during and after giving birth. Some neighborhoods we serve have some of the highest rates of infant death in the state. We are working to move this needle away from mortality and toward vitality. Since the inception, Show Me Strong Families has supported nearly 1,000 birthing families. We still have more work to do.

On a personal level, I was raised in a family of three girls, one with a high birth success rate. My eldest sister gave birth to nine children. My mother and I (the youngest) both experienced two miscarriages, and my middle sister delivered two still-born babies between two healthy births, which framed my expectations about pregnancy. I vividly remember enjoying a late January barbeque and Super Bowl party to celebrate my middle sister's birthday. After enjoying a hearty meal, I was sitting on the couch and my sister sat next to me and placed her hand on my bulging belly. After a few seconds she said, "You just had a contraction." I said, "No, it's just my food digesting." She said, "No, that was a contraction." She kept her hand on my belly and said, "They're coming pretty close together. We should go to the hospital." I did not feel anything, but did what she told me to do. We headed to the hospital. My physician at the time was the former chief of obstetrics and was out of town. I was swiftly admitted for a three-day stay in the hospital (I was indeed having frequent contractions). I underwent a frightening amniocentesis test to measure the strength of my baby's heart and lungs. They insert a "giant" needle directly into your stomach while you are awake and encourage you not to move. Three days later, I was sent home and placed on bedrest with a prescription for over-the-counter magnesium. After one month of bed rest, I gave birth to a healthy son 2½ weeks prior to his due date. I still recall begging my physician to let me stay in the hospital a few more days, fearing discharge and being sent home expecting to care for a tiny little human alone while my then-husband worked ten-hour overnight shifts. I enrolled in PAT a few months after my son was born. Nick is now a 30-year-old with a very full beard. My story is filled with uncertainty, fear, and joy.

This book is a platform for both knowledge and stories – like mine. It brings together important research that helps us understand why some mothers and babies face higher risks than others, and it shares the real-life experiences of those who have been through these challenges. By combining these perspectives, we aim to make the issues clearer and more personal, moving beyond statistics to reveal the human stories behind them.

We also highlight the work of those on the front lines – practitioners, community leaders, and advocates – who are finding new ways to support mothers, babies, their families, and communities. Their stories of hope show us what is possible when communities come together to provide care that is compassionate, respectful, and responsive to the unique needs of each family. From programs that bring support directly to homes, to community groups that offer a listening ear and a helping hand, these stories demonstrate what can be done to ensure a safer, healthier journey for mothers, babies, families, and communities.

We hope that this book will be a source of inspiration and practical guidance for those who care about the well-being of mothers, babies, and families. It is a call to action, reminding us that every mother deserves the chance to thrive, and that together, we can create a world where every birth story is one of hope and possibility. Through the stories and knowledge shared here, we invite you to join us in working toward a future where all families can feel safe, supported, and celebrated in their journey through pregnancy and beyond.

PAT is proud to be a part of this book alongside our colleagues from the Brazelton Touchpoints Center. We know that relationships matter and through the trusting relationships that home visitors and other community and service professionals form with families, we together can impact child and family outcomes not only in our community, but in communities across the world.

Constance Gully
President and Chief Executive Officer, Parents as Teachers National Center
St. Louis, Missouri, United States
December 2024

Acknowledgments

This book was made possible through an initiative funded by Parents as Teachers National Center, in partnership with the Brazelton Touchpoints Center.

The authors extend their appreciation to Parents as Teachers' president and chief executive officer, Constance Gully, for writing the Preface; to Amanda Million, for creating the cover artwork; to Stephanie Tian for assisting with the literature review; and to the frontline staff and community service providers that shared their stories (featured throughout the book) of how communities are coming together to address the morbidity and mortality crisis during pregnancy and beyond.

Disclaimers

While this book broadly discusses medical topics, none of its contents should be construed as medical advice. Please consult a medical professional with questions and concerns.

The stories of several pregnant and postpartum individuals and families are shared throughout this book. Several of these stories were gathered by the authors, who received permission to include them in the book with names and identifying details changed (denoted with a Δ throughout the book). Others are stories which have been widely publicized in news media by the affected individuals and/or their loved ones; in these cases, names and identifying details have not been altered, in keeping with what has been publicly reported (denoted with a ∞ throughout the book). Others are amalgams of personal and publicly available stories (denoted with a ♥ throughout the book).

Correspondence

Please address general correspondence to Christina F. Mondi, Ph.D. (Christina.Mondi-Rago@childrens.harvard.edu). Please address any correspondence related to Parents as Teachers specifically to Allison Kemner, MPH (Allison.Kemner@parentsasteachers.org).

1 Introduction to Pregnancy and Birth-Related Health Outcomes

Self-Care Moment

The topic of this book is heavy. Yet, it is important to stay grounded in hope and the reasons we do this work. Before reading this chapter, close your eyes and think back on your work with families. Call to mind a peaceful or happy moment between a parent and their baby (or recall a happy moment with another baby you know). Recall the joy in their eyes, the smiles on their faces, and the connection between them. Hold this moment in your mind as you read this book.

In recent years, tragic stories of deaths during pregnancy and the postpartum period have gained increased attention, spotlighting the critical gaps in healthcare that affect people of all backgrounds. From well-known figures to everyday parents, these losses underscore the vulnerability of childbirth and the urgent need for systemic change. Celebrities like Beyoncé and Serena Williams have shared their own near-death experiences, highlighting that pregnancy-related health crises transcend fame and wealth. Meanwhile, stories from news outlets reveal the heartbreaking realities faced by other families, particularly in communities of color where pregnancy- and birth-related health complications and death rates are disproportionately high. By sharing these experiences, this book honors those who have suffered and those who have lost their lives and urges a collective response to improve outcomes for all families.

Key Terms

Parent: Any adult who plays a primary caregiving role in a child's life, including but not limited to: biological parents; step, foster, or adoptive parents; caregiving grandparents, etc.

Family: Individuals who care about and/or are closely connected to a child, including but not limited to: biological, step, foster, or adoptive family (immediate or extended); chosen family, etc.

DOI: 10.4324/9781003476474-1

Maria's Story Δ

Maria's story is one of strength and resilience, but it also highlights the harsh realities that many individuals – particularly those of color – face in the healthcare system during and after pregnancy.

Maria is a 32-year-old Latina living in a predominantly low-income neighborhood in the heart of Phoenix, Arizona. She and her husband were thrilled to find out that she was pregnant with their first child. As a first-generation American, Maria had grown up seeing her parents work tirelessly to provide for their family. Now, she wanted to ensure her baby had every opportunity for a healthy start. However, Maria's pregnancy journey was marked by a series of complications and systemic challenges that ultimately turned a joyful time into one fraught with fear and uncertainty.

Prenatal Care: Facing Barriers From the Start

From the beginning of her pregnancy, Maria struggled to access consistent prenatal care. Living in an area with few obstetricians and an overburdened community clinic, she had difficulty scheduling her first appointment until her second trimester. When she finally met with her healthcare provider, Maria noticed that the staff seemed rushed and detached, making her feel more like a number than a patient. She tried to ask questions about her health and the baby's development, but often received curt, incomplete answers.

Language also became a significant barrier. While Maria is bilingual, her husband is not. The lack of Spanish-language materials and interpreters during some visits left them both feeling confused and anxious. When Maria mentioned persistent back pain and extreme fatigue, these concerns were dismissed as "normal pregnancy symptoms," despite the fact that she knew something felt off. Maria's concerns were not thoroughly investigated until later, when it was discovered that she had gestational diabetes – a condition that could have been detected and managed much earlier with appropriate screening and communication.

Birth: A Traumatic Experience

When Maria went into labor, she arrived at the hospital feeling hopeful but was soon confronted with another layer of challenges. As a Medicaid (public health insurance) recipient, she felt the subtle but palpable difference in the way she was treated compared to other people in the labor and delivery unit. The hospital was understaffed, and nurses came in sporadically, leaving Maria alone and frightened for long stretches of time. Despite reporting intense pain and decreased fetal movement, she was not taken seriously by providers.

It was not until several hours later that a nurse realized that the baby was in distress. Maria was rushed for an emergency Cesarean section (C-section) delivery. When her son was delivered, he needed to be resuscitated and transferred to the neonatal intensive care unit (NICU) for breathing complications. For Maria, the joy of her son's birth was overshadowed by guilt and fear. She could not help but wonder if more attentive care could have prevented this crisis.

Postpartum: Isolation and Unmet Needs

The difficulties did not end after Maria and her son were discharged from the hospital. She had developed postpartum preeclampsia, a dangerous condition that causes high blood pressure and can lead to strokes if left untreated. Maria had severe headaches and swelling, but she postponed going to the hospital because she feared the medical bills and worried that her symptoms would once again be dismissed. Her husband had taken time off work to help care for her, but without paid leave, their finances were becoming strained.

When Maria finally went to the emergency room, she felt scrutinized and judged rather than supported. She was asked questions about her diet, her adherence to prenatal appointments, and even her citizenship status – all of which made her feel as though she were to blame for her condition. It was only after a second blood pressure spike that a compassionate nurse stepped in and ensured that Maria received the care she needed.

Social and Structural Factors at Play

Maria's story is not an isolated one. The complications she faced were exacerbated by social and structural factors that shape the healthcare experiences of many families of color. Limited access to quality prenatal care, implicit bias in treatment, language barriers, and lack of culturally sensitive care all contributed to the challenges Maria faced.

Maria's neighborhood is a designated "obstetric care desert," with few providers and long wait times at the local clinic. Her experience with Medicaid, while providing some healthcare access, was marred by stigma and insufficient coverage for additional services that could have been helpful, such as lactation consultation or mental health support. The intersection of her race, gender, and socioeconomic status placed her at a higher risk for the very conditions she experienced, yet the healthcare system was ill-equipped to proactively address these risks.

Every year, more than 134 million babies are born around the world.[1] While the circumstances of these pregnancies and births vary widely, parents and communities everywhere hope that their babies will enter the world safely, in good health, and surrounded by love and support. Unfortunately, an alarming number of individuals – like Maria – are affected by health challenges and complications, and even death during pregnancy, the postpartum period, and the first year of life – with tremendous impacts for them, their families, and their communities in both the short and long terms (and even across generations).[2] This book explores these patterns, with particular attention to the role that community and social service providers, including home visitors, can play in promoting healthy pregnancies and positive birth outcomes for all families, especially those at greatest risk.

Key Terms

Morbidity: Health problems or complications (physical or mental). The term "health problems/complications" will typically be used throughout this book, and the focus will be on health problems/complications related to pregnancy and/or childbirth.

Mortality: Death. This book discusses mortality that is related to the circumstances of pregnancy, childbirth, and/or postpartum recovery.

Well-being: A state of physical and mental health, happiness, and good functioning in everyday life.

Prenatal period: Pregnancy, which runs 40 weeks if carried to full-term. In medical terms, pregnancy is tracked and dated based on the first day of the last menstrual period. In cases of natural conception, the menstrual period is followed by ovulation (when an ovary releases an egg, about two weeks post-menstruation) and fertilization (when egg and sperm meet, forming a zygote). Thus, at the time of fertilization, a person is already considered to be "two weeks pregnant."

Fetus: The medical term for the unborn offspring that is growing inside a uterus. The term "fetus" is used starting nine weeks after fertilization until birth.

Postpartum period: The 12-month (one year) period after giving birth.

Newborn: A delivered baby, from birth through two or three months of age.

Infant: A delivered baby, from birth through 12 months (one year) of age.

Pregnancy- and Birth-Related Health Problems/Complications and Death

Despite medical advances, more than a quarter of a million individuals around the world died from pregnancy or birth-related health problems/complications in 2020, with most of those deaths occurring due to preventable causes.[3] Most of these deaths occurred in low-income regions of the world (e.g., sub-Saharan Africa, Southern Asia), with an average rate of 430 deaths per 100,000 live births in low-income countries.[3] Death rates are much lower in most high-income countries with an average of 12 pregnant or postpartum individuals dying per 100,000 live births – with the notable exception of the United States, where 33 pregnant or postpartum individuals die for every 100,000 live births.[3,4] While death is the ultimate tragedy, it is also important to acknowledge that for every death, there are many others who experience adverse but non-fatal health problems.[5]

Take Time to Reflect

When did you first become aware of how common health problems/complications and death are during pregnancy, the postpartum period, and the first year of life? What information or events brought this to your attention (i.e., events in your personal or family life, professional experiences, news or media stories)?

Recent estimates have also indicated that each year over two million newborns around the world die within the first month of life, and that twice as many die within the first year of life – with most deaths occurring in low-income regions.[6,7] In the United States, the infant mortality rate was about 56 deaths per one million live births in 2022.[8] Millions of other infants experience non-fatal health problems/complications during pregnancy, childbirth, and/or the first year of life.

Disparities in Health Outcomes

Certain groups are at particularly high risk for adverse outcomes related to pregnancy and childbirth – for example, people of color, those with low socioeconomic resources, those who identify as LGBTQ+, and those with disabilities. Notably, non-Hispanic Black women and American Indian and Alaska Native women in the United States are three and two times more likely, respectively, to die from pregnancy-related causes than White women.[9] These patterns are related to persistent bias and socioeconomic disparities in the United States, both within healthcare systems and in communities at large. Similar patterns are also evident in many other regions across the world.

Behind every statistic are people and stories. In recent years, a growing number of individuals and families have publicly shared their experiences of health problems/complications, death, and discrimination during and after pregnancy.[10,11,12,13,14] These include celebrities like tennis champion Serena Williams,[15] singer-songwriter Beyoncé,[16] former National Football League cheerleader Krystal Anderson,[17] and former Olympic athletes Allyson Felix[18] and Tori Bowie.[19] They also include medical professionals like pediatric resident Dr. Chaniece Williams[20] and NICU nurse Lauren Bloomstein.[21] These stories and so many others highlight the pervasiveness of discrimination and disparities even at high levels of socioeconomic, educational, and occupational advantage. They also reflect countless stories that are not publicized in the media, including, perhaps, those of your neighbors, friends, or family – or even yourself.

The Role of Community and Social Service Providers

As public awareness around pregnancy and birth-related health problems, complications, and death has grown, the United States and many other countries have announced numerous initiatives and investments intended to improve health outcomes.[22] Many of these initiatives have been geared toward medical professionals (i.e., obstetrician/gynecologists, nurses, midwives) and have focused on improving safety during childbirth. This work is extremely important. However, research has identified the following three key facts which point to a need for additional types and timing of support.

1. Most incidents of health problems/complications and death during pregnancy, the postpartum period, and the first year of life are preventable.
2. Many of the individual-level risk and protective factors for health problems, complications, and death are present before a pregnancy is even conceived (e.g., pre-pregnancy health conditions, health literacy and self-advocacy skills, substance use).
3. There are many social and structural determinants of health (SDOH) – i.e., non-medical, environmental, structural conditions – that affect pregnancy outcomes and that contribute to disparities (Figure 1.1).

Each of these points listed will be discussed in depth later in this book. Taken together, they underscore the importance of providing early, ongoing, and multi-dimensional support as

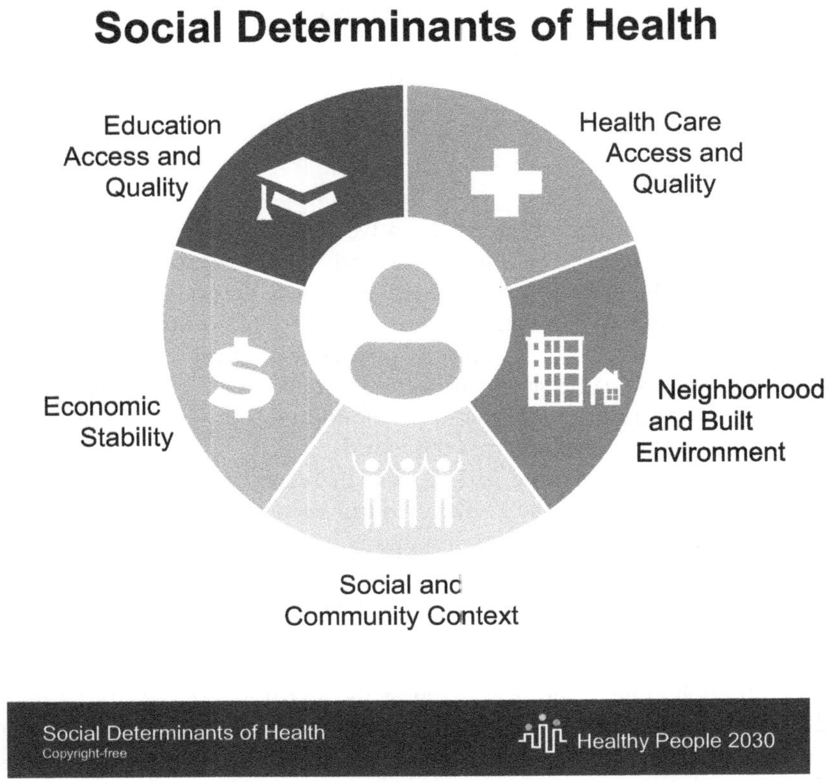

Figure 1.1 Social determinants of health (SDOH) from *Healthy People 2030* (U.S. Department of Health and Human Services)

Note: This copyright-free graphic from the U.S. Department of Health and Human Services[23] highlights five key SDOH categories: (a) economic stability (i.e., employment opportunities and living wages, food and housing costs); (b) education access and quality (i.e., reading and math skills, high school graduation rates); (c) healthcare access and quality (i.e., access to preventive medical care and screenings for children and adults, access to publicly funded contraceptive services, access to care in one's language); (d) neighborhood and built environment (i.e., internet access, exposure to toxic pollutants, access to smoke-free environments); and (e) social and community context (i.e., community connectedness, supports for caregivers of people with disabilities). Later chapters of this book will explore all these categories as they specifically relate to pregnancy, the postpartum period, and the first year of life.

people navigate family planning, pregnancy, and the postpartum period. This level of support is beyond most healthcare providers' scope of work with families, but *is* well within the scope of work for many community and social service providers – the audience and focus of this book.

Examples of Community and Social Service Providers

- Home visitors
- Community health workers (i.e., community health representatives, peer mentors or navigators, care coordinators, public health workers)

- Health education specialists
- Social workers
- Doulas
- Therapists and counselors
- Parent educators

The Role of Community and Social Service Providers

Community and social service providers like you have significant potential to reduce rates of health problems/complications and death during pregnancy, the postpartum period, and the first year of life. Consider the work that you (or someone you know) has done with families during these times in their lives. What conversations did you have? What experiences did they share with you? What knowledge did you share? What concerns did they lift up?

As someone who interacts with families in their homes or in the community, you often get to know their lives in great detail – what their strengths and stressors are, what household and community resources they do and do not have access to, and much more. The relationships that you form with families can be ideal avenues for sharing critical health information, for creating safe spaces to develop and practice self-advocacy skills, and for following up to ensure that they have access to needed resources. You may be the most trusted provider they have, and the one with whom they feel most comfortable sharing important and sensitive social and health information. Ultimately, whatever the topic and strategy, your strongest tool to support families during pregnancy and the postpartum period is your relationship with them.

Maria's Story Continued: Raising Awareness and A Call to Action Δ

Maria's story sheds light on the health crisis that disproportionately affects people of color and their babies in the United States. To improve outcomes, we must address the SDOH that create barriers to care and contribute to preventable complications. Doing so includes training healthcare, community, and social service providers to recognize and counteract implicit biases, and ensuring that all families have access to the support and healthcare that they need – regardless of their income, race, or citizenship status. By listening to and elevating stories like Maria's, we can work toward a healthcare system that honors every family's experience and ensures a healthy start for every baby.

About This Book

We, the authors, are a diverse group of practitioners (parent educators, home visitors, psychologists, nurse practitioners), researchers, and public health experts who are passionate about supporting the well-being of infants, children, families, and communities. Some of us are based out of the Parents as Teachers National Center (PATNC), the headquarters most known for the Parents as Teachers (PAT) evidence-based home visiting model that is used around the world. Others are based out of the Research and Evaluation Unit at the Brazelton Touchpoints Center (BTC), part of the Division of Developmental Medicine at Boston Children's Hospital. For several years, our teams have been collaborating on a multi-phase project aimed at: (a) understanding the experiences of pregnant and postpartum families in home visiting (drawing on decades of published research, as well as original research and evaluation activities with hundreds of home visitors and families); and (b) developing and testing new strategies for reducing disparities and promoting well-being among these groups.

The work together of PATNC and BTC has been deep and rewarding, and it has resulted in many valuable insights and resources for PAT affiliates and families – and yet, we recognize that the problems of adverse pregnancy- and birth-related health outcomes go far beyond the communities that PAT serves. As noted earlier in this chapter, we have also come to realize that most existing resources and research on these topics are geared toward professionals who work in healthcare settings. Thus, we have compiled this book with community and social service providers in mind, with the intention of accessibly and usefully presenting wisdom from both research and practice that these providers can apply to their work with pregnant and postpartum families.

Our approach to writing this book was strongly guided by a bioecological perspective, which recognizes that human development and well-being is affected by many factors (i.e., biology, the family, support networks; broader social, cultural, and community conditions).[24] We also aim to take a strengths-based approach that highlights individual, family, and community assets, strengths, and opportunities in addition to any risk factors or stressors. Throughout, we have also endeavored to embody a spirit of self-reflection and cultural humility on our part as an author team.

Table 1.1 provides an outline for the remainder of the book. Chapters 2–9 include stories, research, and reflection questions, as well as specific strategies related to the individual topics within each chapter. These strategies will generally fall into one of a few categories: (a) sharing knowledge; (b) building skills; and (c) strengthening self-efficacy. While the specific strategies may vary, these are the foundational elements of your role that we believe can make the biggest impact. Throughout, we will also encourage you to think about your role not only as a service provider for individual families, but as an ambassador and advocate for issues that affect the families you work with.

A Note About Descriptions of Study Samples

When describing research study findings throughout this book, we have aimed to describe samples using the same language used in the original study manuscript (i.e., regarding race/ethnicity and other factors).

A Note About Medical Advice

Importantly, as previously noted, this book is geared toward professionals working with pregnant and postpartum families in community and social service – not healthcare – settings. Although we will broadly discuss health and healthcare challenges, nothing in this book should be construed as medical advice, and families should always be directed to speak with a trusted healthcare professional about any individual health questions or concerns.

Table 1.1 Outline of Remaining Book Chapters

Chapter	*Topics Covered*
Chapter 2: Physical Health Problems and Complications During Pregnancy, the Postpartum Period, and the First Year of Life	Physical health problems and complications during pregnancy and the postpartum period (i.e., gestational diabetes, hypertension, preeclampsia, hemorrhage) and affects on their babies (i.e., atypical birthweight, preterm birth, traumatic brain injury), with a focus on risk and protective factors that could be addressed via preventive healthcare, community-based interventions, and/or public policy.
Chapter 3: Mental Health During Pregnancy and the Postpartum Period	Mental health (i.e., depression, anxiety) during pregnancy and the postpartum period, with a focus on risk and protective factors that could be addressed via preventive healthcare, community-based interventions, and/or public policy.
Chapter 4: Substance Use During Pregnancy and the Postpartum Period	Substance use (i.e., opioid use, tobacco use) during pregnancy and the postpartum period, with a focus on risk and protective factors that could be addressed via preventive healthcare, community-based interventions, and/or public policy.
Chapter 5: Death During Pregnancy, the Postpartum Period, and the First Year of Life	Death during pregnancy, the postpartum period, and the first year of life, with particular focus on risk and protective factors that could be addressed via preventive healthcare, community-based interventions, and/or public policy.
Chapter 6: Healthcare During the Preconception Period and Pregnancy	The importance of accessing high-quality, responsive healthcare early and often during the preconception and prenatal periods, with particular focus on the role that community and social service providers can play in addressing disparities in healthcare access among the populations they serve.
Chapter 7: Healthcare During Childbirth and the Postpartum Period	The importance of accessing high-quality, responsive healthcare during childbirth and the postpartum period, with particular focus on the role that community and social service providers can play in addressing disparities in healthcare access among the populations they serve.
Chapter 8: Healthcare and Breastfeeding During the First Year of Life	The importance of high-quality, culturally sensitive healthcare for newborns and infants in the first year of life, with particular focus on the role that community and social service providers can play in addressing disparities in healthcare access among the populations they serve. The chapter also discusses benefits, disparities, and interventions related to breastfeeding.
Chapter 9: Supporting Healthy Lifestyles and Relationships	Lifestyle and relationship factors that have been shown to affect health and well-being during pregnancy and the postpartum period (i.e., nutrition, exercise, sleep), with particular focus on the role that community and social service providers can play in addressing disparities and supporting healthy lifestyles and relationships among the populations they serve.
Chapter 10: Synthesis and Call to Action	A final call for community and social service providers to join the fight to improve pregnancy and birth-related outcomes in their local communities.

Key Takeaways From This Chapter

1. Around the world, far too many people experience preventable health problems/complications, and even death. In many regions, certain groups are at particularly high risk – for example, people of color, those with low socioeconomic resources, those who identify as LGBTQ+, and those with disabilities.

2. Many of the individual-level risk and protective factors for health problems, complications, and death are present before a pregnancy is even conceived. There are also many SDOH (i.e., non-medical, environmental, and/or structural conditions) that affect health outcomes and disparities.
3. The relationships that community and social service providers form with families can be ideal avenues for sharing critical health information, for creating safe spaces to develop and practice self-advocacy skills, and for following up to ensure that they have access to needed resources.

References

1. UNICEF (n.d.). *How many babies are born a year?* https://data.unicef.org/how-many/how-many-babies-are-born-a-year/
2. Kozhimannil, K. B. (2018). Reversing the rise in maternal mortality. *Health Affairs, 37*(11). https://doi.org/10.1377/hlthaff.2018.1013
3. World Health Organization (WHO) (2023). *Maternal mortality.* www.who.int/news-room/fact-sheets/detail/maternal-mortality#:~:text=A%20woman's%20lifetime%20risk%20of,49%20in%20low%2Dincome%20countries
4. Joseph, K. S., Lisonkova, S., Boutin, A., Muraca, G. M., Razaz, N., John, S., Sabr, Y., Chan, W., Mehrabadi, A., Brandt, J. S., Schisterman, E. F., & Ananth, C. V. (2024). Maternal mortality in the United States: Are the high and rising rates due to changes in obstetrical factors, maternal medical conditions, or maternal mortality surveillance? *Obstetrics, 230*(4), 440.e1–440.e13. https://doi.org/10.1016/j.ajog.2023.12.038
5. World Health Organization (WHO) (2024a). *Maternal morbidity and well-being.* www.who.int/teams/maternal-newborn-child-adolescent-health-and-ageing/maternal-health/maternal-morbidity-and-well-being
6. World Health Organization (WHO) (2024b). *Infant mortality.* www.who.int/data/gho/data/themes/topics/indicator-groups/indicator-group-details/GHO/infant-mortality
7. World Health Organization (WHO) (2024c). *Newborn mortality.* www.who.int/news-room/fact-sheets/detail/newborn-mortality#:~:text=There%20are%20approximately%206500%20newborn,to%202.3%20million%20in%202022.
8. Ely, D. M., & Driscoll, A. K. (2023). Infant mortality in the United States: Provisional data from the 2022 period linked birth/infant death file. *Vital Statistics Rapid Release, 33.* www.cdc.gov/nchs/data/vsrr/vsrr033.pdf. Accessed December 2024.
9. Hill, L., Artiga, S., & Ranji, U. (2022). Racial disparities in maternal and infant health: Current status and efforts to address them. *Racial Equity and Health Policy.* www.kff.org/racial-equity-and-health-policy/issue-brief/racial-disparities-in-maternal-and-infant-health-current-status-and-efforts-to-address-them/
10. Centers for Disease Control and Prevention (2023). *HEAR HER campaign.* www.cdc.gov/hearher/index.html. Accessed December 2024.
11. Green, E. L. (2023, January 18). "I don't want to die": Fighting maternal mortality among black women. *The New York Times.* www.nytimes.com/2023/01/18/us/doula-black-women.html
12. Miller, C. C., Kliff, S., & Buchanan, L. (2023, February 12). Childbirth is deadlier for black families even when they're rich, expansive study finds. *The New York Times.* www.nytimes.com/interactive/2023/02/12/upshot/child-maternal-mortality-rich-poor.html
13. ProPublica (2024). *Lost mothers: Maternal care and preventable deaths.* www.propublica.org/series/lost-mothers
14. The Lullaby Trust (n.d.). *"When my baby died": Parents tell their stories.* www.lullabytrust.org.uk/wp-content/uploads/15-parents-stories.pdf
15. Williams, S. (2022, April 5). How Serena Williams saved her own life. *Elle.* www.elle.com/life-love/a39586444/how-serena-williams-saved-her-own-life/
16. FitzPatrick, H. (2019, April 18). Beyoncé opens up about pregnancy complications with twins. *ABC News.* https://abcnews.go.com/GMA/Culture/beyonce-opens-pregnancy-complications-twins/story?id=62480855#:~:text=%22I%20was%20218%20pounds%20the,an%20emergency%20C%2Dsection.%22

17. Calvario, L. (2024, March 26). Longtime Kansas City Chiefs cheerleader Krystal Anderson dies after giving birth. *NBC News.* www.nbcnews.com/health/womens-health/longtime-kansas-city-chiefs-cheerleader-krystal-anderson-dies-giving-b-rcna145221
18. Centers for Disease Control and Prevention (2022). *Unexpected pregnancy complications: Allyson Felix's story.* www.cdc.gov/hearher/allysonfelix/index.html#:~:text=She%20never%20imagined%20that%20she,in%20an%20emergency%20C%2Dsection. Accessed December 2024.
19. Chappell, B. (2023). Tori Bowie, an elite Olympic athlete, died of complications from childbirth. *NPR.* www.npr.org/2023/06/13/1181971448/tori-bowie-an-elite-olympic-athlete-died-of-complications-from-childbirth
20. Washington, T. (2020). Death of young mother brings attention to racial differences in maternal mortality. *WRTV.* www.wrtv.com/news/working-for-you/death-of-young-mother-brings-attention-to-racial-differences-in-maternal-mortality
21. Martin, N., ProPublica, & Montagne, R. (2017). The last person you'd expect to die in childbirth. *ProPublica.* www.propublica.org/article/die-in-childbirth-maternal-death-rate-health-care-system
22. The White House (2024, July 10). *The White House blueprint for addressing the maternal health crisis: Two years of progress.* www.whitehouse.gov/briefing-room/statements-releases/2024/07/10/the-white-house-blueprint-for-addressing-the-maternal-health-crisis-two-years-of-progress/. Accessed December 2024.
23. U.S. Department of Health and Human Services, Office of Disease Prevention and Health Promotion (n.d.). *Healthy People 2030.* https://health.gov/healthypeople/objectives-and-data/social-determinants-health. Accessed December 2024.
24. Bronfenbrenner, U. (1977). Toward an experimental ecology of human development. *American Psychologist, 32*(7), 513–531. https://doi.org/10.1037/0003-066X.32.7.513

2 Physical Health Problems and Complications During Pregnancy, the Postpartum Period, and the First Year of Life

> **Self-Care Moment**
>
> Reading about health problems/complications can be difficult, particularly if you or someone you know are currently pregnant or previously had a difficult pregnancy. Before diving into this chapter, take a few deep, cleansing breaths – in through your nose like you are smelling a flower, and out through your mouth like you are blowing out birthday candles.

Pregnancy is truly a multi-month marathon. Researchers have found that during pregnancy, the body works as hard as in an extreme athletic event, like an ultramarathon or the Tour de France.[1] To this end, even pregnancies without complications come with a range of physical symptoms and changes (see Table 2.1).

Table 2.1 Examples of Common Physical Symptoms During Pregnancy[2,3,4]

First Trimester	• Nausea, vomiting, and food aversions • Fatigue • Breast tenderness and swelling • Bloating, mild cramping, and light spotting • Increased urination • Constipation
Second Trimester	• Mild contractions • Skin changes • Congestion and other nasal problems • Sensitive teeth and gums • Dizziness • Leg cramps • Vaginal discharge • Urinary tract infections
Third Trimester	• Mild contractions • Back and pelvic pain • Shortness of breath • Heartburn • Hemorrhoids • Increased urination

(*Continued*)

DOI: 10.4324/9781003476474-2

Table 2.1 (Continued)

First Trimester	• Nausea, vomiting, and food aversions • Fatigue • Breast tenderness and swelling • Bloating, mild cramping, and light spotting • Increased urination • Constipation
Postpartum	• Vaginal soreness (after a vaginal delivery) • Pain and tenderness around the incision site (after a C-section) • Vaginal discharge • Contractions • Hemorrhoids • Urine leakage • Breast tenderness • Hair loss • Skin changes

It can be difficult to determine which of the physical changes and symptoms outlined in Table 2.1 are "normal" and which may be of concern. Therefore, it is important during pregnancy to be aware of typical symptoms, potential warning signs of more serious health problems/complications, and where to turn for help.[5] As an integral part of families' support network during and after pregnancy, it is also important for you to be informed about these topics, so that you can help them identify and access the healthcare or support services that they need.

This chapter focuses on preventing, identifying, and responding to physical health problems/complications (also known as *morbidities*) during pregnancy, the postpartum period, and the first year of life, including a discussion of research on this topic, practice implications for your work, and reflections on your role as a community or social service provider. Throughout this chapter, you will also hear the stories of Sarah and Cam, two mothers living in very different communities who each faced serious physical health complications following the birth of their children.

Sarah's Story, Part 1 Δ

Sarah's story is one of resilience in the face of both the joys and unexpected perils of parenthood. Her journey began with a lifelong dream: to become a mother. Sarah had already experienced a miscarriage before the birth of her first child and was living in a rural community in Illinois, nearly an hour's drive away from the hospital.

Cam's Story, Part 1 Δ

Cam was living with her partner and toddler in a large metropolitan area when she learned that she was pregnant with their second child. Her story highlights the importance of paying close attention to physical symptoms, listening to one's instincts, and advocating for healthcare attention.

Research Summary and Implications for Community and Social Service Providers

> **Key Terms**
>
> **Gestational diabetes**: A form of diabetes (high blood sugar disorder) that is diagnosed for the first time during pregnancy. Gestational diabetes is a serious condition which, if left untreated, can lead to serious or even fatal outcomes. These include hypertension and preeclampsia, preterm birth, need for C-section, breathing difficulties in the newborn, and stillbirth.
>
> **Hypertension**: High blood pressure. If left untreated, hypertension can lead to serious or even fatal outcomes such as preeclampsia, stroke, and placental abruption (separation of the placenta from the uterine wall).
>
> **Preeclampsia**: A serious health condition during pregnancy or the postpartum period related to high blood pressure that often involves bodily swelling and urination changes, among other symptoms. When left untreated, preeclampsia can lead to serious or even fatal outcomes such as seizures, kidney or liver failure, and blood clotting.

New-Onset Health Problems/Complications During Pregnancy

In some cases, physical health problems/conditions are present before pregnancy; in others, new problems/conditions develop for the first time during pregnancy. Two of the most common health problems/complications that can arise during pregnancy are: (a) gestational diabetes; and (b) hypertension and preeclampsia.[6] Notably, both gestational diabetes and hypertension often have few initial obvious symptoms and are only detected through health screenings – underscoring the importance of regular prenatal care.

Diabetes

According to the U.S. Centers for Disease Control and Prevention (CDC),[7] approximately 8% of pregnancies in the United States were affected by gestational diabetes in 2021. This rate was nearly six times higher among mothers who were 40 years or older compared to those who were 20 years or younger. Researchers have also found that pregnant women of color are at significantly higher risk of developing gestational diabetes compared to non-Hispanic White women, as are those living in poverty and those who have relatively lower levels of education.[8,9,10] Pre-pregnancy obesity and weight gain in between pregnancies have also been linked to increased risk of developing gestational diabetes.[11,12]

Diagnosis and management of gestational diabetes is typically a multi-stage process. Screening for gestational diabetes typically occurs between 24 and 28 weeks of a pregnancy as a standard part of prenatal care, but can occur sooner if additional risk factors are present (for example, obesity prior to pregnancy; having a biological parent, sibling, or child with diabetes; or having had gestational diabetes in a prior pregnancy). Screening begins with an initial glucose challenge test. If the results suggest gestational diabetes, a follow-up glucose tolerance test will be conducted to confirm the diagnosis. These tests both consist of drinking a glucose drink and testing the levels of glucose in the body after one- and three-hour intervals.

Patients who have been diagnosed with gestational diabetes may experience a range of emotions (such as worrying about their baby's health or how they will manage additional medical bills), as well as a steep learning curve to understand the disease and how to manage it.[13,14,15,16] Researchers have found that those who have recently been diagnosed with gestational diabetes often feel that their healthcare providers have done a poor job of explaining information to them, and struggle to make lifestyle changes and to participate in follow-up healthcare.[16,17,18]

Researchers have also identified several important protective factors and potential interventions for patients with gestational diabetes. These include: (a) providing clear, concrete, and culturally relevant education on pregnancy planning and healthy lifestyles during pregnancy; (b) encouraging reflection on one's goals for themselves, their babies, and their families; and (c) increasing access to social support.[19,20,21,22] Community and social service providers can play significant roles in supporting the development of these protective factors for those who have gestational diabetes or who are at risk for developing it.

Hypertension and Preeclampsia

According to the CDC,[23] approximately 16% of pregnancies in the United States were affected by hypertensive disorders at the time of delivery. Significantly higher rates of hypertensive disorders have been found among Black and Indigenous mothers and other women of color, those affected by poverty and other stressors, those living in rural areas, those living in socioeconomically disadvantaged areas, those giving birth at older ages, and those diagnosed with obesity or diabetes.[12,23,24,25,26,27,28,29,30] In a large study in California, researchers found that higher socioeconomic status reduced the risk for preeclampsia among White women, but not Black women – pointing to the disparities and barriers that Black people face at all socioeconomic levels.[24]

As with gestational diabetes, the diagnosis and treatment process for hypertension and preeclampsia is often lengthy and complicated – including blood tests, urine tests, and tracking of symptoms. In a focus group study, many women who had experienced preeclampsia reported that their healthcare provider did a poor job explaining the disorder and how to manage it, and that social support played an important role in helping them cope.[31] As with gestational diabetes, community and social service providers, including home visitors, can play significant roles in supporting those who have hypertension and/or preeclampsia, or who are at risk for these conditions.

Putting It Into Practice

- ***Discuss family planning as a standard part of services with all families.*** Many of the risk and protective factors for prenatal health problems/complications are present before a pregnancy is even conceived, making family planning and preconception health very important topics. Further, spacing between births affects pregnancies, parenting, and family well-being. Initiate these conversations by acknowledging the potential sensitivity of the topic and asking families if they are open to having a conversation about their pregnancy plans, desires, and/or visions for their family size.

- ***Learn about the individual's health status, including pre-pregnancy health issues.*** Many risk and protective factors for health are present before a pregnancy is even conceived, and those who have pre-existing health conditions are at increased risk for health complications during pregnancy. Have ongoing conversations with your clients about their physical and mental health at a level at which they are comfortable. Explore how their health connects to the health of their baby.
- ***Support the development of protective factors for those who have gestational diabetes or who are at risk for developing it.*** As mentioned previously, researchers have identified several valuable interventions that providers can implement with pregnant clients who are at risk for gestational diabetes or who have been diagnosed with it. These include: (a) providing clear, concrete, and culturally relevant education on pregnancy planning and maintaining a healthy lifestyle; (b) encouraging them to reflect on their goals for themselves, their babies, and their families; and (c) increasing their access to social support.[19,20,21,22] You can help reinforce and process information they are receiving about gestational diabetes and support them in setting specific, incremental, and measurable goals related to managing their condition. You may also be able to refer expecting parents to support groups of others in similar situations.
- ***Provide timely information about physical and social and emotional changes during pregnancy, as well as fetal development.*** As a community or social service provider, you likely meet with parents more frequently and for longer periods than healthcare providers do. This extended period of time and relationship creates an opportunity for parents to process information at their own pace, formulate questions, and make plans for follow-up. Your supportive relationship can be of particular benefit for those experiencing pregnancy and postpartum complications as they process symptoms, information, and emotional reactions.

Take Time to Reflect

Think about your role supporting pregnant families. How might you approach a conversation with a family around pregnancy symptoms and what is considered typical? What might your next steps be if they describe or recognize a symptom you think may indicate gestational diabetes or hypertension?

Severe Maternal Health Problems/Complications Around the Time of Labor and Delivery

Sarah's Story, Part 2 Δ

Sarah gave birth to her first child at the hospital, and at first, everything seemed to go flawlessly. Then, shortly after delivering the baby, Sarah suddenly began to experience excessive and uncontrolled internal bleeding – severe postpartum hemorrhage. Her medical team initially thought she might need a blood transfusion but was ultimately able to manage the situation and to discharge Sarah two days after she gave birth. This unexpected crisis clouded Sarah's early days of motherhood with fear and confusion. No one had warned her about the medical complications that could arise after a healthy pregnancy and textbook delivery. Sarah felt lucky to still be alive and able to have more children, but the sense of betrayal by her own body never really escaped her.

Eight years later, when Sarah and her husband, Ben, welcomed their fourth and final child, another challenge loomed. After returning home from the hospital, Sarah noticed some unusual postpartum symptoms, such as reduction in breastmilk supply, intense cramping, and light vaginal bleeding with unusual (large) blood clotting. She messaged her medical team, but they initially dismissed her concerns. By the time Sarah finally received an ultrasound 26 days after giving birth, it was discovered that a piece of placenta had been retained in her uterus after the delivery and had become infected. Her doctor scheduled her for a procedure to remove the retained placenta, which should have been a routine outpatient surgery. However, during the surgery, an instrument punctured Sarah's uterus (which was already weakened by infection), causing life-threatening internal bleeding. Sarah's condition quickly escalated to an emergency situation and she had to undergo a hysterectomy (removal of the uterus) – a step that she and her husband never imagined would become necessary, especially with Sarah only being 32 years old. Ben felt unprepared and overwhelmed by the life-altering decisions that he had to make as Sarah's power of attorney while she was under anesthesia and feared that he might never speak to his wife again. Sarah's condition stabilized after the procedure, but the effects of this event were long-lasting.

Cam's Story, Part 2 Δ

A few days after giving birth to her second child and returning home from the hospital, Cam felt extremely fatigued and noticed swelling in her ankles and feet. Cam called her doctor who said she was probably fine and just needed to rest. As Cam hung up the phone, she noticed that her head was starting to ache, too. "Am I overblowing this?" she wondered. "The doctor said I'm probably fine, but I just don't feel right."

Cam was worried, but she wasn't sure what to do next. Then she thought of her home visitor, Shonda, with whom she had been working for over a year. During their last home visit before giving birth, Shonda had encouraged her to reach out anytime with concerns or questions.

Cam picked up the phone again, called Shonda, and told her what was going on. Shonda listened carefully. She urged Cam to trust her gut and go to the emergency room to get checked out. There, Cam learned that she was experiencing a serious condition called postpartum preeclampsia. The doctor said that if she had not gone to the emergency room, she could have suffered very serious health complications or even died.

Key Term

Severe maternal morbidity (SMM), or, severe maternal health problems/complications: "Unexpected outcomes of labor and delivery that result in significant short- or long-term consequences to . . . health."[32]

SMM includes serious physical health complications, most of which occur around the time of labor and delivery. Clinicians and researchers do not fully agree on what conditions should be counted under the umbrella of SMM,[33] but the following box lists examples identified by the CDC. Even if you are not a medical professional, it is important to have some knowledge of the types of SMM that can affect the pregnant and postpartum clients you work with, particularly if risk factors and warning signs are left unidentified or untreated.

CDC 's 21 Indicators of SMM (Severe Maternal Health Problems or Complications) During Childbirth Hospitalizations[34]

- Acute myocardial infarction (heart attack)
- Aneurysm
- Acute renal failure (acute kidney failure)
- Acute respiratory distress syndrome
- Amniotic fluid embolism (when amniotic fluid or other fetal materials enter the birthing person's bloodstream, blocking blood supply)
- Cardiac arrest (sudden loss of heart activity)/ventricular fibrillation (irregular heartbeat)
- Conversion of cardiac rhythm (medical procedure to reestablish a normal heartbeat)
- Disseminated intravascular coagulation (a disorder involving overactive blood clotting)
- Blood transfusion
- Eclampsia (new-onset seizures)
- Heart failure/arrest during surgery or procedure
- Puerperal cerebrovascular disorders (disorders involving blood flow and vessels in the brain)

- Pulmonary edema (excessive fluid in the lungs)/acute heart failure
- Severe anesthesia complications
- Sepsis (a serious reaction to an infection)
- Shock (a serious reaction to reduced blood flow in the body)
- Sickle cell disease with crisis
- Air and thrombotic embolism (when air bubbles or a blood clot, respectively, block blood supply in the blood vessels or heart)
- Hysterectomy (surgical removal of the uterus)
- Temporary tracheostomy (surgical procedure that creates an opening in the windpipe for breathing)
- Ventilation (breathing with the support of a medical ventilator machine)

Self-Care Moment

You just read a long list of frightening complications that can happen during and after pregnancy. Before you continue, take a moment to take some more deep, cleansing breaths. Breathe in through your nose like you are smelling a flower, and out through your mouth like you are blowing out birthday candles.

Take Action

Take a moment to consider what you would do if you were visiting a pregnant or postpartum client, and they began to experience serious health symptoms (i.e., difficulty breathing, profuse bleeding). What research or basic trainings might be helpful for you and your colleagues? You might consider questions like:

- Do you know how to contact local emergency services?
- Do you know where the nearest emergency department or urgent care center is located?
- Do you know how to perform basic first aid and cardiopulmonary resuscitation (CPR)?

During labor and delivery, severe health complications are much more common than death,[35] and alarmingly, research has shown that rates of SMM have increased in recent years.[36] Those with SMM are also more likely to have lengthy hospital stays after giving birth, and to be readmitted not long after initial discharge.[37,38,39]

Black and Indigenous mothers and other mothers of color are more likely to experience SMM than White mothers in the United States and many other countries.[40,41,42,43,44,45,46,47,48,49,50,51,52] This remains true for those giving birth at the same hospital and even after accounting for co-occurring health problems, C-section delivery, and other factors.[40] These patterns suggest that systematic inequities may contribute to heightened rates of SMM among mothers of color. For example, in the United States and many other settings, people of color are more likely to face social and economic stressors which may affect their health and well-being (i.e., racism, poverty, lack of access to culturally appropriate healthcare). Healthcare providers may not adequately address warning signs or risk factors for SMM among their pregnant patients of color due to implicit bias, lack of cultural understanding, limited resources, or other factors.[53] These issues will be discussed further throughout this book.

Across racial and ethnic groups, the warning signs and risk and protective factors for SMM are often present long before labor begins. For example, researchers have found that the following person-level factors are associated with increased risk of SMM.

- Young maternal age (younger than 20 years)[54] or advanced maternal age (35 years or older);[40,55,56,57,58,59]
- Co-occurring physical health conditions (i.e., pregnancy-related hypertension, human immunodeficiency virus [HIV] infection, chronic physical disabilities);[40,48,60,61,62,63,64,65]
- Intellectual or developmental disability;[66]
- Co-occurring mental health conditions, such as depression or bipolar disorder;[54]
- Having public insurance (i.e., Medicaid) versus private or employer-based insurance;[44]
- Lack of prenatal care;[44]
- Hospitalization prior to pregnancy;[52]
- Being hospitalized early in pregnancy;[44]
- Excessive weight gain during pregnancy;[67]
- Being pregnant with multiples;[44]
- Giving birth early;[44] and
- History of SMM in previous pregnancies.[68,69]

Researchers have also identified hospital- and community-level factors that are associated with increased risk of severe health complications, including the following.

- Structural racism in the local area (i.e., racial inequalities in female educational attainment);[70]
- High levels of poverty in the local area;[54]
- Living in an area where the local hospitals are poorly rated;[54] and
- Giving birth in a hospital that serves a high proportion of patients of color.[35]

Putting It Into Practice

- ***Learn about local healthcare providers.*** Develop a working knowledge of capable and responsive healthcare providers. This knowledge is often invaluable in helping families to navigate complex healthcare systems.
- ***Validate the family's concerns and questions during the prenatal and postpartum periods, supporting them in bringing these to a healthcare provider.*** Pregnancy and the postpartum period can be times of great uncertainty and many questions. Many individuals may feel shut down by prior negative experiences or are hesitant to bring forward concerns. Strive to create environments and relationships in which individuals and family members feel safe in bringing forward

concerns and questions. Coaching, roleplaying, and practice are all strategies that can be used to help clients prepare for healthcare visits and consultations.

- ***Discuss with the family what typically occurs during childbirth and consider options for support and advocacy in the place where they will be giving birth.*** Feeling informed can contribute to being more comfortable, calm, and capable, all of which can help make for a positive birthing experience. During childbirth, it can be especially helpful to have the support and potential advocacy of trusted family members, friends, or a doula. Help your pregnant clients identify who these people are for them. Help families to navigate making specific requests of their circle of support – both things they would like them to be prepared to do on their behalf and things they would like them to refrain from during and after the birth.
- ***Facilitate the development of a birthing plan.*** Some pregnant clients find it helpful to put together a written birth plan that clarifies how they would ideally like to approach labor and delivery. You can support them in reflecting on their preferences, locating and completing a birth plan template, and sharing the plan with their healthcare provider. It is also important to discuss the potential need for flexibility in the plan depending on how the pregnancy and childbirth process unfold.
- ***Check in with the family in the days following delivery.*** The first days at home following a birth can be emotional and stressful, on top of the experience of physically recovering from giving birth. During these early days, parents and families may be especially receptive to assistance from those with whom they already have established, trusting relationships. During this time, offer emotional support and connections to critical resources like lactation consultation. Encourage parents to follow-up with healthcare providers about any health concerns or symptoms for themselves or their newborn.
- ***Encourage attendance at least one postpartum visit with a healthcare provider.*** Postpartum healthcare is an essential part of the physical recovery process, particularly if there were any health complications along the way. However, attending these appointments can often feel difficult for new parents who are navigating overnight wakings, transportation challenges, childcare needs for other children, and more. Share information with families about the benefits of postpartum healthcare and help them to make plans to attend that feel manageable.

Physical Health Problems/Complications Among Infants

Sarah's Story, Part 3 Δ

The trauma of Sarah's and Ben's experiences did not end in the hospital. The couple's newborn had contracted respiratory syncytial virus (RSV) and pneumonia from visiting Sarah in the intensive care unit (ICU), leading to yet another hospital stay for the family. Juggling physical and emotional recovery with the demands of motherhood and supporting her family became overwhelming, affecting Sarah's marriage and mental health.

Key Terms

Preterm birth: When birth occurs before 37 weeks gestation. Preterm birth is associated with increased risk of health problems for the newborn, such as neurodevelopmental conditions, breathing and feeding difficulties, vision and hearing problems, and death.

Atypical birthweight and/or size for gestational age: When a newborn is significantly smaller or bigger than expected based on when they were delivered (i.e., gestational age). Newborns who are smaller than expected are at increased risk for breathing, feeding, and temperature regulation difficulties, neurological and gastrointestinal problems, sudden infant death syndrome (SIDS), and more. Newborns who are larger than expected are at increased risk for injury during birth, breathing problems and low blood sugar shortly after birth, and more. Both conditions are also associated with increased risk of long-term health problems.

Unfortunately, physical health problems and complications also affect newborns and infants. The complications for newborns and infants often go hand in hand with maternal health and well-being. Two of the most commonly occurring physical health complications among infants are: (a) preterm birth; and (b) atypical birthweight and/or size for gestational age. It is important for community and social service providers to have some knowledge of these health complications so that they can effectively support affected families.

Preterm Birth

According to the March of Dimes,[71] approximately 1 in 10 births in the United States occurred preterm in 2022. Preterm birth can be caused by a combination of genetic factors, environmental factors, and/or social disparities. Higher rates of preterm birth have been documented among infants of color, as well as those whose mothers were underweight or obese before getting pregnant, had physical or mental health problems, were intellectually disabled, had significant stressors (including worry about racial discrimination), and/or had less time between pregnancies, among other factors.[12,36,61,72,73,74,75,76,77,78,79,80,81,82,83,84,85] Research has also found that racism at the community level (i.e., institutional policies, racial/ethnic segregation) is associated with increased risk of preterm birth.[86,87] One study found that Black infants from areas with higher uninsurance rates among Black adults, fewer Black physicians, and fewer publicly funded family planning services were more likely to be born preterm.[88]

There have been several protective factors and potential strategies identified for preventing preterm birth across groups. Notably, in one study, parents who had experienced preterm birth reported wanting the following.

- "Power in knowledge and control" related to their healthcare; and
- Thoughtfully chosen information (including information about medical risk and options), presented in sensitive, easy-to-understand, and empowering ways[89 (p.E9)]

Timely prenatal care has also been found to be a protective factor related to preterm birth.[90]

Atypical Birthweight and/or Size for Gestational Age

At the time of delivery, weight and/or size that is either much lower or higher than typical can have negative health implications, though much of the research has focused on the lower end of the size spectrum. Researchers have found that babies whose mothers are people of color are more likely to be born small for gestational age compared to infants of White mothers, as are babies who are born to parents who are older, have public insurance, have limited prenatal care, have physical or mental health problems, have many stressors, and/or are underweight or obese before pregnancy.[12,55,56,73,77,78,84,91,92,93,94,95,96]

Regarding protective factors, researchers have found that father/partner involvement in pregnancy is associated with lower risk of low birthweight, and that infants whose parents receive a community health worker or home visiting services are also less likely to be born at a low birthweight. Timely prenatal care has also been identified as a protective factor for reducing rates of low birthweight.[97]

Putting It Into Practice

- ***Work with all parents and caregivers in the family.*** Father/partner involvement in pregnancy is associated with decreased risk of negative outcomes for mothers and babies. Families may also have multiple parents or caregivers (i.e., step-parents), and/or multigenerational care structures. Whereas healthcare providers typically focus their attention on their pregnant patient, community and social service providers are often well positioned to work with the entire family system. This approach recognizes families' realities as dynamic and interconnected and can lead to better outcomes.
- ***Ask families about the timing of their baby's birth, and their baby's size at birth.*** Families with babies who were preterm, small for gestational age, or large for gestational age may benefit from additional support, particularly if baby is experiencing any ongoing health problems/complications.

Your Role as a Community or Social Service Provider

Listening and Learning

The data and information in this chapter present a picture of the physical challenges that can arise during and after pregnancy. Understanding the data and statistics specific to your community will help you to tailor your services to the issues, needs, and strengths of your local community and the families within it. Consider: what do you already know about the physical health complications that pregnant families in your local community experience (i.e., how often they occur, which types of complications are most common)? How can you learn more?

In addition to researching local data and statistics, you can also make a difference by listening to personal stories of families in your community. You can then use these stories to tailor and improve the services that you and your colleagues offer, so that they are culturally appropriate and genuinely responsive to the needs of your community. Consider: how can you connect with more pregnant and postpartum families in your area and hear their stories, opinions, and ideas?

Advocating

Your role as a community or service provider can be seen as operating on two levels: (a) your individual work with families, and (b) your work with systems. Both individual- and systems-level work are important. Individual work with families can help families live within and navigate systems in a way that is most beneficial to them. Consider: what is one example of how your work with families has helped them navigate a system in a way that has been beneficial to them?

At the same time, it is important to work with system representatives to make comprehensive changes that will prevent and reduce physical health problems/complications during and after pregnancy. The systems level includes local healthcare, housing, education, transportation, human services, and more. Your organization's established connections with these systems can facilitate families' access to needed and desired services and resources. Further, connections with systems provide avenues for broader advocacy. Coordinating with system representatives and leaders can result in positive change for many in your community. Consider: what is an example of system advocacy you have engaged in? What kind of system advocacy would you like to be involved in?

Cam's Story, Part 3 Δ

The relationship that Cam had with her home visitor Shonda and the way that Shonda validated her health concerns helped save her life. With medical attention, Cam made a full recovery. She and her family continued to participate in home visiting services, and over time she grew in knowledge and confidence in her roles as a self-advocate and parent.

Sarah's Story, Part 4 Δ

With support from extended family and a new therapist, Sarah and Ben made it through this stressful and traumatic time for their family. They rebuilt their connection, improved their communication, and found new ways to better support each other as partners and parents.

Outside of the home, Sarah had a job as a parent educator, working with parents of young children. Ultimately, her labor and postpartum experiences became a wellspring of empathy and purpose. She often found herself wondering, "What if this had happened to a family I work with?" These words became her guiding light, and she used her experiences to shape her work with families by offering an understanding that only someone who has been through the depths of maternal health complications can provide. Her journey propelled her into leadership roles where she could make an even larger impact – becoming a supervisor before ultimately joining PATNC, supporting programs across the world in implementing home visiting programs that can change the lives of families during pregnancy, the postpartum period, kindergarten, and beyond.

Sarah's hope is to foster open communication about maternal health problems/ complications and death through sharing her story so that no one else feels unheard or ashamed for facing similar struggles. Her story serves as a rallying cry for families, healthcare providers, and advocates to address maternal health problems/complications openly and proactively. She has dedicated her life to helping others find hope and strength in the face of adversity, knowing that her own story has given her the power to make a difference.

Take Time to Reflect

Reflecting on the practice implications throughout this chapter and your role as a community or social service provider, what is one area where you believe you are already doing an excellent job? What is one area where you could improve your professional practice or deepen your learning and understanding?

Take Action

Now that you have reflected on an area where you could improve your professional practice, create a SMART goal to make it happen, described as follows.

- **S**pecific
- **M**easurable
- **A**chievable
- **R**elevant
- **T**ime-Bound

For example, imagine that you would like deepen your practice around working with multiple parents or caregivers in the family system, not just the pregnant client. A SMART goal might be:

> Many of the pregnant families I work with are made up of multigenerational households and/or have co-parents (**Relevant**). By the end of this year (**Time-Bound**), I will intentionally increase my interactions with those people, so that I am interacting with family members or co-parents for at least 50% of my caseload (**Measurable, Specific, Achievable**). I will track my progress and interactions with different family members in my caseload spreadsheet.

As you create your own SMART goals, think about how you might also use this strategy to support the goal-setting of families you work with.

Key Takeaways From This Chapter

1. Some of the most common physical health conditions that can arise during pregnancy are gestational diabetes, hypertension, and preeclampsia. For babies, preterm birth

and atypical birthweight and/or size for gestational age are among the most common complications.

2. Some groups are more likely to experience physical health complications during and after pregnancy (i.e., people of color, low-income people). This is largely due to barriers in accessing high-quality healthcare, as well as other SDOH.
3. Community and social service providers can take many steps to promote physical well-being during and after pregnancy, even if they are not in the healthcare field. The relationships that they build with families over time put them in a strong position to make a difference.

References

1. Thurber, C., Dugas, L. R., Ocobock, C., Carlson, B., Speakman, J. R., & Pontzer, H. (2019). Extreme events reveal an alimentary limit on sustained maximal human energy expenditure. *Science Advances*, *5*(6), eaaw0341. https://doi.org/10.1126/sciadv.aaw0341
2. Mayo Clinic Staff (2024, February 27). 1st trimester pregnancy: What to expect. *Mayo Clinic.* https://www.mayoclinic.org/healthy-lifestyle/pregnancy-week-by-week/in-depth/pregnancy/art-20047208
3. Mayo Clinic Staff (2025, February 7). 2nd trimester pregnancy: What to expect. *Mayo Clinic.* https://www.mayoclinic.org/healthy-lifestyle/pregnancy-week-by-week/in-depth/pregnancy/art-20047732
4. Mayo Clinic Staff (2025, February 7). 3rd trimester pregnancy: What to expect. *Mayo Clinic.* https://www.mayoclinic.org/healthy-lifestyle/pregnancy-week-by-week/in-depth/pregnancy/art-200467675
5. Vladutiu, C. J., Stringer, E. M., Kandasamy, V., Ruppenkamp, J., & Menard, M. K. (2019). Emergency care utilization among pregnant Medicaid recipients in North Carolina: An analysis using linked claims and birth records. *Maternal and Child Health Journal*, *23*(2), 265–276. https://doi.org/10.1007/s10995-018-2651-6
6. Harris, A., Chang, H. Y., Wang, L., Sylvia, M., Neale, D., Levine, D., & Bennett, W. (2015). Emergency room utilization after medically complicated pregnancies: A Medicaid claims analysis. *Journal of Women's Health*, *24*(9), 745–754. https://doi.org/10.1089/jwh.2014.5125
7. U.S. Centers for Disease Control and Prevention (2023). *QuickStats:* Percentage of mothers with gestational diabetes, by maternal age – National Vital Statistics System, United States, 2016 and 2021. *MMWR Morbidity and Mortality Weekly Report*, *72*(16). https://doi.org/10.15585/mmwr.mm7201a4. Accessed December 2024.
8. Bower, J. K., Butler, B. N., Bose-Brill, S., Kue, J., & Wassel, C. L. (2019). Racial/ethnic differences in diabetes screening and hyperglycemia among US women after gestational diabetes. *Preventing Chronic Disease*, *16*. http://doi.org/10.5888/pcd16.190144
9. Liu, B., Lamerato, L. E., & Misra, D. P. (2020). A retrospective analysis of the relationship between race/ethnicity, age at delivery and the risk of gestational diabetes mellitus. *The Journal of Maternal-Fetal & Neonatal Medicine*, *33*(17), 2961–2969. https://doi.org/10.1080/14767058.2019.1566310
10. Wilson, B. L., Dyer, J. M., Latendresse, G., Wong, B., & Baksh, L. (2015). Exploring the psychosocial predictors of gestational diabetes and birth weight. *Journal of Obstetric, Gynecologic & Neonatal Nursing*, *44*(6), 760–771. https://doi.org/10.1111/1552-6909.12754
11. Lynes, C., McLain, A. C., Yeung, E. H., Albert, P., Liu, J., & Boghossian, N. S. (2017). Interpregnancy weight change and adverse maternal outcomes: A retrospective cohort study. *Annals of Epidemiology*, *27*(10), 632–637. https://doi.org/10.1016/j.annepidem.2017.09.008
12. Shin, D., & Song, W. O. (2015). Prepregnancy body mass index is an independent risk factor for gestational hypertension, gestational diabetes, preterm labor, and small-and large-for-gestational-age infants. *The Journal of Maternal-Fetal & Neonatal Medicine*, *28*(14), 1679–1686. https://doi.org/10.3109/14767058.2014.964675
13. Carolan-Olah, M., Duarte-Gardea, M., Lechuga, J., & Salinas-Lopez, S. (2017). The experience of gestational diabetes mellitus (GDM) among Hispanic women in a US border region. *Sexual & Reproductive Healthcare*, *12*, 16–23. https://doi.org/10.1016/j.srhc.2016.11.003

14. Craig, L., Sims, R., Glasziou, P., & Thomas, R. (2020). Women's experiences of a diagnosis of gestational diabetes mellitus: A systematic review. *BMC Pregnancy and Childbirth*, *20*(1), 76. https://doi.org/10.1186/s12884-020-2745-1
15. McCloskey, L., Quinn, E., Ameli, O., Heeren, T., Craig, M., Lee-Parritz, A., Iverson, R., Jack, B., & Bernstein, J. A. (2019). Interrupting the pathway from gestational diabetes mellitus to type 2 diabetes: The role of primary care. *Women's Health Issues*, *29*(6), 480–488. https://doi.org/10.1016/j.whi.2019.08.003
16. Oza-Frank, R., Conrey, E., Bouchard, J., Shellhaas, C., & Weber, M. B. (2018). Healthcare experiences of low-income women with prior gestational diabetes. *Maternal and Child Health Journal*, *22*(7), 1059–1066. https://doi.org/10.1007/s10995-018-2489-y
17. Bernstein, J. A., McCloskey, L., Gebel, C. M., Iverson, R. E., & Lee-Parritz, A. (2016). Lost opportunities to prevent early onset type 2 diabetes mellitus after a pregnancy complicated by gestational diabetes. *BMJ Open Diabetes Research and Care*, *4*(1), e000250. http://doi.org/10.1136/bmjdrc-2016-000250
18. Werner, E. F., Has, P., Kanno, L., Sullivan, A., & Clark, M. A. (2019). Barriers to postpartum glucose testing in women with gestational diabetes mellitus. *American Journal of Perinatology*, *36*(2), 212–218. http://doi.org/10.1055/s-0038-1667290
19. Athavale, P., Thomas, M., Delgadillo-Duenas, A. T., Leong, K., Najmabadi, A., Harleman, E., Rios, C., Quan, J., Soria, C., & Handley, M. A. (2016). Linking high risk postpartum women with a technology enabled health coaching program to reduce diabetes risk and improve wellbeing: Program description, case studies, and recommendations for community health coaching programs. *Journal of Diabetes Research*, *2016*. https://doi.org/10.1155/2016/4353956
20. McGrath, M., & Chrisler, J. C. (2017). A lot of hard work, but doable: Pregnancy experiences of women with type-1 diabetes. *Health Care for Women International*, *38*(6), 571–592. https://doi.org/10.1080/07399332.2016.1267183
21. Yee, L. M., McGuire, J. M., Taylor, S. M., Niznik, C. M., & Simon, M. A. (2016). Factors promoting diabetes self-care among low-income, minority pregnant women. *Journal of Perinatology*, *36*(1), 13–18. https://doi.org/10.1038/jp.2015.134
22. Yee, L. M., Niznik, C. M., & Simon, M. A. (2016). Examining the role of health literacy in optimizing the care of pregnant women with diabetes. *American Journal of Perinatology*, *33*(13), 1242–1249. http://doi.org/10.1055/s-0036-1584540
23. Ford, N. D., Cox, S., Ko, J. Y., Ouyang, L., Romero, L., Colarusso, T., Ferre, C. D., Kroelinger, C. D., Hayes, D. K., & Barfield, W. (2022). Hypertensive disorders in pregnancy and mortality at delivery hospitalization – United States, 2017–2019. *MMWR Morbidity and Mortality Weekly Report*, *71*(17). Accessed December 2024.
24. Hitti, J., Sienas, L., Walker, S., Benedetti, T. J., & Easterling, T. (2018). Contribution of hypertension to severe maternal morbidity. *American Journal of Obstetrics and Gynecology*, *219*(4), 405-e1. https://doi.org/10.1016/j.ajog.2018.07.002
25. Hux, V. J., & Roberts, J. M. (2015). A potential role for allostatic load in preeclampsia. *Maternal and Child Health Journal*, *19*(3), 591–597. https://doi.org/10.1007/s10995-014-1543-7
26. Levine, L. D., Nkonde-Price, C., Limaye, M., & Srinivas, S. K. (2016). Factors associated with postpartum follow-up and persistent hypertension among women with severe preeclampsia. *Journal of Perinatology*, *36*(12), 1079–1082. https://doi.org/10.1038/jp.2016.137
27. Ren, M., Li, H., Cai, W., Niu, X., Ji, W., Zhang, Z., Niu, J., Zhou, X., & Li, Y. (2018). Excessive gestational weight gain in accordance with the IOM criteria and the risk of hypertensive disorders of pregnancy: A meta-analysis. *BMC Pregnancy and Childbirth*, *18*(1), 1–9. https://doi.org/10.1186/s12884-018-1922-y
28. Ross, K. M., Schetter, C. D., McLemore, M. R., Chambers, B. D., Paynter, R. A., Baer, R., Feuer, S. K., Flowers, E., Karasek, D., Pantell, M., Prather, A. A., Ryckman, K., & Jelliffe-Pawlowski, L. (2019). Socioeconomic status, preeclampsia risk and gestational length in black and white women. *Journal of Racial and Ethnic Health Disparities*, *6*(6), 1182–1191. https://doi.org/10.1007/s40615-019-00619-3
29. Ruhstaller, K. E., Bastek, J. A., Thomas, A., Mcelrath, T. F., Parry, S. I., & Durnwald, C. P. (2016). The effect of early excessive weight gain on the development of hypertension in pregnancy. *American Journal of Perinatology*, *33*(12), 1205–1210. http://doi.org/10.1055/s-0036-1585581

30. Lemon, L. S., Hauspurg, A., Garrard, W., Quinn, B., & Simhan, H. N. (2023). Neighborhood disadvantage and the racial disparity in postpartum hypertension. *American Journal of Obstetrics & Gynecology MFM*, *5*(1), 100773. https://doi.org/10.1016/j.ajogmf.2022.100773
31. Skurnik, G., Roche, A. T., Stuart, J. J., Rich-Edwards, J., Tsigas, E., Levkoff, S. E., & Seely, E. W. (2016). Improving the postpartum care of women with a recent history of preeclampsia: A focus group study. *Hypertension in Pregnancy*, *35*(3), 371–381. https://doi.org/10.3109/10641955.2016.1154967
32. U.S. Centers for Disease Control and Prevention (2023). *Severe maternal morbidity*. www.cdc.gov/maternal-infant-health/php/severe-maternal-morbidity/?CDC_AAref_Val=www.cdc.gov/reproductivehealth/maternalinfanthealth/severematernalmorbidity.html. Accessed December 2024.
33. Kilpatrick, S. J., Abreo, A., Gould, J., Greene, N., & Main, E. K. (2016). Confirmed severe maternal morbidity is associated with high rate of preterm delivery. *American Journal of Obstetrics and Gynecology*, *215*(2), 233-e1. http://doi.org/10.1016/j.ajog.2016.02.026
34. U.S. Centers for Disease Control and Prevention (2023). *Identifying severe maternal morbidity (SMM)*. www.cdc.gov/maternal-infant-health/php/severe-maternal-morbidity/icd.html. Accessed December 2024.
35. Howell, E. A., Egorova, N., Balbierz, A., Zeitlin, J., & Hebert, P. L. (2016). Black-white differences in severe maternal morbidity and site of care. *American Journal of Obstetrics and Gynecology*, *214*(1), 122-e1. https://doi.org/10.1016/j.ajog.2015.08.019
36. Leonard, S. A., Main, E. K., & Carmichael, S. L. (2019). The contribution of maternal characteristics and cesarean delivery to an increasing trend of severe maternal morbidity. *BMC Pregnancy and Childbirth*, *19*(1), 1–9. http://doi.org/10.1186/s12884-018-2169-3
37. Clapp, M. A., Little, S. E., Zheng, J., & Robinson, J. N. (2016). A multi-state analysis of postpartum readmissions in the United States. *American Journal of Obstetrics and Gynecology*, *215*(1), 113-e1. http://doi.org/10.1097/01.AOG.0000483643.12760.91
38. Girsen, A. I., Sie, L., Carmichael, S. L., Lee, H. C., Foeller, M. E., Druzin, M. L., & Gibbs, R. S. (2020). Rate and causes of severe maternal morbidity at readmission: California births in 2008–2012. *Journal of Perinatology*, *40*(1), 25–29. https://doi.org/10.1038/s41372-019-0481-z
39. Van Otterloo, L., Connelly, C., Gould, J., Abreo, A., & Main, E. (2018). Mothers at risk: Factors affecting maternal postpartum length of stay. *The Journal of Perinatal & Neonatal Nursing*, *32*(4), 303–314. http://doi.org/10.1097/JPN.0000000000000342
40. Aziz, A., Gyamfi-Bannerman, C., Siddiq, Z., Wright, J. D., Goffman, D., Sheen, J. J., D'Alton, M. E., & Friedman, A. M. (2019). Maternal outcomes by race during postpartum readmissions. *American Journal of Obstetrics and Gynecology*, *220*(5), 484.e1–484.e10. https://doi.org/10.1016/j.ajog.2019.02.016
41. Booker, W. A., Gyamfi-Bannerman, C., Sheen, J. J., Wright, J. D., Siddiq, Z., D'Alton, M. E., & Friedman, A. M. (2018). Maternal outcomes by race for women aged 40 years or older. *Obstetrics and Gynecology*, *132*(2), 404–413. https://doi.org/10.1097/AOG.0000000000002751
42. Harper-Hanigan, K., Ross, G., Sims, T., Trotter, K., & Turman, J. E., Jr (2017). Women's perspectives of needs surrounding adverse birth outcomes: A qualitative assessment of the neighborhood impact of adverse birth outcomes. *Maternal and Child Health Journal*, *21*(12), 2219–2228. https://doi.org/10.1007/s10995-017-2343-7
43. Howell, E. A., Egorova, N. N., Shondavic, T., Brodman, M., Balbierz, A., Zeitlin, J., & Hebert, P. L. (2020a). Race and ethnicity, medical insurance, and within-hospital severe maternal morbidity disparities. *Obstetrics and Gynecology*, *135*(2), 285–293. https://doi.org/10.1097/AOG.0000000000003667
44. Howell, E. A., Shondavic, T., Blum, J., Zeitlin, J., Egorova, N. N., Balbierz, A., & Hebert, P. L. (2020b). Double disadvantage in delivery hospital for black and Hispanic women and high-risk Infants. *Maternal and Child Health Journal*, *24*(6), 687–693. https://doi.org/10.1007/s10995-020-02911-9
45. Johnson, P. D., Duzyj, C. M., Howell, E. A., & Shondavic, T. (2019). Patient and hospital characteristics associated with severe maternal morbidity among postpartum readmissions. *Journal of Perinatology*, *39*(9), 1204–1212. https://doi.org/10.1038/s41372-019-0426-6
46. Leonard, S. A., Crespi, C. M., Gee, D. C., Zhu, Y., & Whaley, S. E. (2015). Prepregnancy risk factors for preterm birth and the role of maternal nativity in a low-income, Hispanic population. *Maternal and Child Health Journal*, *19*(10), 2295–2302. https://doi.org/10.1007/s10995-015-1748-4

47. Parchem, J. G., Gupta, M., Chen, H. Y., Wagner, S., Mendez-Figueroa, H., & Chauhan, S. P. (2020). Adverse infant and maternal outcomes among low-risk term pregnancies stratified by race and ethnicity. *Obstetrics and Gynecology, 135*(4), 925–934. https://doi.org/10.1097/AOG.0000000000003730
48. Martin, J., Croteau, A., Velasco-Gonzalez, C., Gastanaduy, M., Huttner, M., Saeed, R., Niazi, S., Chisholm, S., Mussarat, N., Morgan, J., Williams, F. B. W., & Biggio, J. (2022). Maternal early warning criteria predict postpartum severe maternal morbidity and mortality after delivery hospitalization discharge: A case-control study. *American Journal of Obstetrics & Gynecology MFM, 4*(6), 100706. https://doi.org/10.1016/j.ajogmf.2022.100706
49. Barreto, T., Li, C., Chung, Y. K., Jabbarpour, Y., Baltrus, P., & Gaglioti, A. (2022). Measuring state-level racial inequity in severe maternal morbidity in the Medicaid population. *Maternal and Child Health Journal, 26*(4), 682–690. https://doi.org/10.1007/s10995-021-03192-6
50. Garg, B., Hersh, A., Caughey, A. B., & Pilliod, R. A. (2022). Severe maternal morbidity and Black-white differences in Washington state. *The Journal of Maternal-Fetal & Neonatal Medicine, 35*(25), 5949–5956. https://doi.org/10.1080/14767058.2021.1903423
51. Leonard, S. A., Main, E. K., Lyell, D. J., Carmichael, S. L., Kennedy, C. J., Johnson, C., & Mujahid, M. S. (2022). Obstetric comorbidity scores and disparities in severe maternal morbidity across marginalized groups. *American Journal of Obstetrics & Gynecology MFM, 4*(2), 100530. https://doi.org/10.1016/j.ajogmf.2021.100530
52. Meadows, A. R., Cabral, H., Liu, C. L., Cui, X., Amutah-Onukagha, N., Diop, H., & Declercq, E. R. (2023). Preconception and perinatal hospitalizations as indicators of risk for severe maternal morbidity in primiparas. *American Journal of Obstetrics & Gynecology MFM, 5*(7), 101014. https://doi.org/10.1016/j.ajogmf.2023.101014
53. Petersen, E. E., Davis, N. L., Goodman, D., Cox, S., Syverson, C., Seed, K., Shapiro-Mendoza, C., Callaghan, W. M., & Barfield, W. (2019). Racial/ethnic disparities in pregnancy-related deaths – United States, 2007–2016. *MMWR Morbidity and Mortality Weekly Report, 68*, 762–765. https://doi.org/10.15585/mmwr.mm6835a3. Accessed December 2024.
54. Reid, L. D., & Creanga, A. A. (2018). Severe maternal morbidity and related hospital quality measures in Maryland. *Journal of Perinatology, 38*(8), 997–1008. https://doi.org/10.1038/s41372-018-0096-9
55. Arya, S., Mulla, Z. D., & Plavsic, S. K. (2018). Outcomes of women delivering at very advanced maternal age. *Journal of Women's Health, 27*(11), 1378–1384. https://doi.org/10.1089/jwh.2018.7027
56. Creanga, A. A., Syverson, C., Seed, K., & Callaghan, W. M. (2017). Pregnancy-related mortality in the United States, 2011–2013. *Obstetrics and Gynecology, 130*(2), 366–373. https://doi.org/10.1097/AOG.0000000000002114
57. Sheen, J. J., Huang, Y., Andrikopoulou, M., Wright, J. D., Goffman, D., D'Alton, M. E., & Friedman, A. M. (2020). Maternal age and preeclampsia outcomes during delivery hospitalizations. *American Journal of Perinatology, 37*(1), 44–52. http://doi.org/10.1055/s-0039-1694794
58. Sheen, J. J., Wright, J. D., Goffman, D., Kern-Goldberger, A. R., Booker, W., Siddiq, Z., D'Alton, M. E., & Friedman, A. M. (2018). Maternal age and risk for adverse outcomes. *American Journal of Obstetrics and Gynecology, 219*(4), 390-e1. https://doi.org/10.1016/j.ajog.2018.08.034
59. Carr, R. C., McKinney, D. N., Cherry, A. L., & Defranco, E. A. (2022). Maternal age-specific drivers of severe maternal morbidity. *American Journal of Obstetrics & Gynecology MFM, 4*(2), 100529. https://doi.org/10.1016/j.ajogmf.2021.100529
60. Arab, K., Spence, A. R., Czuzoj-Shulman, N., & Abenhaim, H. A. (2017). Pregnancy outcomes in HIV-positive women: A retrospective cohort study. *Archives of Gynecology and Obstetrics, 295*(3), 599–606. https://doi.org/10.1007/s00404-016-4271-y
61. Clements, K. M., Mitra, M., Zhang, J., & Iezzoni, L. I. (2016). Pregnancy characteristics and outcomes among women at risk for disability from health conditions identified in medical claims. *Women's Health Issues, 26*(5), 504–510. https://doi.org/10.1016/j.whi.2016.06.001
62. Guglielminotti, J., Landau, R., Wong, C. A., & Li, G. (2019). Patient-, hospital-, and neighborhood-level factors associated with severe maternal morbidity during childbirth: A cross-sectional study in New York State 2013–2014. *Maternal and Child Health Journal, 23*(1), 82–91. https://doi.org/10.1007/s10995-018-2596-9
63. Iezzoni, L. I., Yu, J., Wint, A. J., Smeltzer, S. C., & Ecker, J. L. (2015). Health risk factors and mental health among US women with and without chronic physical disabilities by whether

women are currently pregnant. *Maternal and Child Health Journal*, *19*(6), 1364–1375. https://doi.org/10.1007/s10995-014-1641-6

64. Lazariu, V., Nguyen, T., McNutt, L. A., Jeffrey, J., & Kacica, M. (2017). Severe maternal morbidity: A population-based study of an expanded measure and associated factors. *PLoS One*, *12*(8), e0182343. https://doi.org/10.1371/journal.pone.0182343
65. Lima, F. V., Parikh, P. B., Zhu, J., Yang, J., & Stergiopoulos, K. (2015). Association of cardiomyopathy with adverse cardiac events in pregnant women at the time of delivery. *JACC: Heart Failure*, *3*(3), 257–266. http://doi.org/10.1016/j.jchf.2014.10.008
66. Mitra, M., Akobirshoev, I., Valentine, A., Brown, H. K., & Moore Simas, T. A. (2021). Severe maternal morbidity and maternal mortality in women with intellectual and developmental disabilities. *American Journal of Preventive Medicine*, *61*(6), 872–881. https://doi.org/10.1016/j.amepre.2021.05.041
67. Platner, M. H., Ackerman, C., Howland, R. E., Xu, X., Pettker, C. M., Illuzzi, J. L., Reddy, U. M., Chung, S., & Lipkind, H. S. (2019). Gestational weight gain and severe maternal morbidity at delivery hospitalization. *Obstetrics & Gynecology*, *133*(3), 515–524. http://doi.org/10.1097/AOG.0000000000003114
68. Bane, S., Wall-Wieler, E., Lyndon, A., & Carmichael, S. L. (2021). Recurrence of severe maternal morbidity: A population-based cohort analysis of California women. *Paediatric and Perinatal Epidemiology*, *35*(2), 155–161. https://doi.org/10.1111/ppe.12714
69. Boulet, S. L., Stanhope, K. K., Worrell, N., & Jamieson, D. J. (2022). Risk of recurrent severe maternal morbidity in an urban safety-net health system. *American Journal of Obstetrics & Gynecology MFM*, *4*(2), 100568. https://doi.org/10.1016/j.ajogmf.2022.100568
70. Liu, S. Y., Fiorentini, C., Bailey, Z., Huynh, M., McVeigh, K., & Kaplan, D. (2019). Structural racism and severe maternal morbidity in New York State. *Clinical Medicine Insights: Women's Health*, *12*, 1179562X19854778. https://doi.org/10.1177/1179562X19854778
71. March of Dimes (2024). *A profile of prematurity in the United States.* www.marchofdimes.org/peristats/reports/united-states/prematurity-profile
72. Almeida, J., Bécares, L., Erbetta, K., Bettegowda, V. R., & Ahluwalia, I. B. (2018). Racial/ethnic inequities in low birth weight and preterm birth: The role of multiple forms of stress. *Maternal and Child Health Journal*, *22*(8), 1154–1163. https://doi.org/10.1007/s10995-018-2500-7
73. Bediako, P. T., BeLue, R., & Hillemeier, M. M. (2015). A comparison of birth outcomes among Black, Hispanic, and Black Hispanic women. *Journal of Racial and Ethnic Health Disparities*, *2*(4), 573–582. https://doi.org/10.1007/s40615-015-0110-2
74. Braveman, P., Heck, K., Egerter, S., Dominguez, T. P., Rinki, C., Marchi, K. S., & Curtis, M. (2017). Worry about racial discrimination: A missing piece of the puzzle of Black-white disparities in preterm birth? *PLoS One*, *12*(10), e0186151. https://doi.org/10.1371/journal.pone.0186151
75. Ferguson, K. K., Rosario, Z., McElrath, T. F., Vélez Vega, C., Cordero, J. F., Alshawabkeh, A., & Meeker, J. D. (2019). Demographic risk factors for adverse birth outcomes in Puerto Rico in the PROTECT cohort. *PLoS One*, *14*(6), e0217770. https://doi.org/10.1371/journal.pone.0217770
76. Koning, S. M., & Ehrenthal, D. B. (2019). Stressor landscapes, birth weight, and prematurity at the intersection of race and income: Elucidating birth contexts through patterned life events. *SSM-Population Health*, *8*, 100460. https://doi.org/10.1016/j.ssmph.2019.100460
77. Shaw, S. H., Herbers, J. E., & Cutuli, J. J. (2019). Medical and psychosocial risk profiles for low birthweight and preterm birth. *Women's Health Issues*, *29*(5), 400–406. https://doi.org/10.1016/j.whi.2019.06.005
78. Teoli, D. A., Zullig, K. J., & Hendryx, M. S. (2015). Maternal fair/poor self-rated health and adverse infant birth outcomes. *Health Care for Women International*, *36*(1), 108–120. https://doi.org/10.1080/07399332.2013.862796
79. Thoma, M. E., Rossen, L. M., De Silva, D. A., Warner, M., Simon, A. E., Moskosky, S., & Ahrens, K. A. (2019). Beyond birth outcomes: Interpregnancy interval and injury-related infant mortality. *Paediatric and Perinatal Epidemiology*, *33*(5), 360–370. https://doi.org/10.1111/ppe.12575
80. Tucker, C. M., Berrien, K., Menard, M. K., Herring, A. H., Daniels, J., Rowley, D. L., & Halpern, C. T. (2015). Predicting preterm birth among women screened by North Carolina's pregnancy medical home program. *Maternal and Child Health Journal*, *19*(11), 2438–2452. https://doi.org/10.1007/s10995-015-1763-5

81. Egbejimi, A., Ajewole, V., Dongarwar, D., Kaur, M., Phillips, M., Liang, J., Fadel, M., Lota, L., Simon, J., Otule, M., Taylor, K., Oguibe, G., Salihu, H. M., & Olaleye, O. (2023). Racial disparities in preterm birth among pregnant women with obesity. *Southern Medical Journal, 116*(6), 471–477. https://doi.org/10.14423/SMJ.0000000000001569
82. Gleason, J. L., Grewal, J., Chen, Z., Cernich, A. N., & Grantz, K. L. (2023). Risk of adverse neonatal outcomes among pregnant women with disabilities. *International Journal of Epidemiology, 52*(1), 203–213. https://doi.org/10.1093/ije/dyac183
83. Boriboonhirunsarn, D., & Tanpong, S. (2023). Rate of spontaneous preterm delivery between pregnant women with and without gestational diabetes. *Cureus, 15*(2), e34565. https://doi.org/10.7759/cureus.34565
84. Elçi, G., Çakmak, A., Elçi, E., & Sayan, S. (2022). The effect of advanced maternal age on perinatal outcomes in nulliparous pregnancies. *Journal of Perinatal Medicine, 50*(8), 1087–1095. https://doi.org/10.1515/jpm-2021-0298
85. Kornfield, S. L., Riis, V. M., McCarthy, C., Elovitz, M. A., & Burris, H. H. (2022). Maternal perceived stress and the increased risk of preterm birth in a majority non-Hispanic Black pregnancy cohort. *Journal of Perinatology, 42*(6), 708–713. https://doi.org/10.1038/s41372-021-01186-4
86. Karvonen, K. L., McKenzie-Sampson, S., Baer, R. J., Jelliffe-Pawlowski, L., Rogers, E. E., Pantell, M. S., & Chambers, B. D. (2023). Structural racism is associated with adverse postnatal outcomes among Black preterm infants. *Pediatric Research, 94*(1), 371–377. https://doi.org/10.1038/s41390-022-02445-6
87. Berkowitz, R. L., Mujahid, M., Pearl, M., Poon, V., Reid, C. K., & Allen, A. M. (2022). Protective places: The relationship between neighborhood quality and preterm births to Black women in Oakland, California (2007–2011). *Journal of Urban Health, 99*(3), 492–505. https://doi.org/10.1007/s11524-022-00624-8
88. Curtis, D. S., Waitzman, N., Kramer, M. R., & Shakib, J. H. (2024). Structural barriers to health care as risk factors for preterm and small-for-gestational-age birth among US-born Black and White mothers. *Health & Place, 85*, 103177. https://doi.org/10.1016/j.healthplace.2024.103177
89. Pizur-Barnekow, K., Kim, U. O., Ahamed, S. I., Dreier, S., Leuthner, S. R., Rau, N., & Basir, M. A. (2020). Giving voice to parents in the development of the Preemie Prep for Parents (P3) mobile app. *Advances in Neonatal Care, 20*(1), E9–E16. http://doi.org/10.1097/ANC.0000000000000669
90. Nasiri, K., Moodie, E. E. M., & Abenhaim, H. A. (2020). Racial disparities in recurrent preterm delivery risk: Mediation analysis of prenatal care timing. *Journal of Perinatal Medicine, 49*(4), 448–454. https://doi.org/10.1515/jpm-2020-0133
91. Guillory, V. J., Lai, S. M., Suminski, R., & Crawford, G. (2015). Low birth weight in Kansas. *Journal of Health Care for the Poor and Underserved, 26*(2), 577–602. http://doi.org/10.1353/hpu.2015.0039
92. Harvey, E. M., Strobino, D., Sherrod, L., Webb, M. C., Anderson, C., White, J. A., & Atlas, R. (2017). Community-academic partnership to investigate low birth weight deliveries and improve maternal and infant outcomes at a Baltimore city hospital. *Maternal and Child Health Journal, 21*(2), 260–266. https://doi.org/10.1007/s10995-016-2153-3
93. Mitra, M., Parish, S. L., Clements, K. M., Cui, X., & Diop, H. (2015). Pregnancy outcomes among women with intellectual and developmental disabilities. *American Journal of Preventive Medicine, 48*(3), 300–308. https://doi.org/10.1016/j.amepre.2014.09.032
94. Davis, K. M., Jones, K. A., Yee, L. M., & Feinglass, J. (2023). Modeling the likelihood of low birth weight: Findings from a Chicago-area health system. *Journal of Racial and Ethnic Health Disparities, 10*(4), 1768–1775. https://doi.org/10.1007/s40615-022-01360-0
95. Huang, D., Liang, M., Xu, B., Chen, S., Xiao, Y., Liu, H., Yin, D., Yang, J., Wang, L., Pan, P., Yang, Y., Zhou, W., & Chen, J. (2023). The association of insufficient gestational weight gain in women with gestational diabetes mellitus with adverse infant outcomes: A case-control study. *Frontiers in Public Health, 11*, 1054626. https://doi.org/10.3389/fpubh.2023.1054626
96. Pollock, E. A., Gennuso, K. P., Givens, M. L., & Kindig, D. (2021). Trends in infants born at low birthweight and disparities by maternal race and education from 2003 to 2018 in the United States. *BMC Public Health, 21*(1), 1117. https://doi.org/10.1186/s12889-021-11185-x
97. Hacker, M., Firk, C., Konrad, K., Paschke, K., Neulen, J., Herpertz-Dahlmann, B., & Dahmen, B. (2021). Pregnancy complications, substance abuse, and prenatal care predict birthweight in adolescent mothers. *Archives of Public Health, 79*(1), 137. https://doi.org/10.1186/s13690-021-00642-z

3 Mental Health During Pregnancy and the Postpartum Period

Self-Care Moment

Before reading this chapter, take a moment to ground yourself by attending to your five senses. What is one thing you can see? Hear? Smell? Taste? Touch? Repeat this exercise a few times while taking deep, calming breaths. This can be a helpful strategy to share when talking about anxiety with a client.

Pregnancy and the postpartum period are often accompanied by changes in nearly every aspect of one's life – from bodily and biological functions to one's sense of personal identity, relationships, routines and responsibilities, and much more. These changes are typically accompanied by a wide range of emotions – from excitement and joy to anxiety and stress. Social support is essential to navigating these shifts and adjusting to this new chapter of life.

In some cases, the stress and emotions that accompany pregnancy and the postpartum period exceed what is typical and move into the realm of more significant mental health challenges (i.e., depression, anxiety, psychosis). In fact, mental health challenges are related to a large number of health complications and deaths during pregnancy and the postpartum period.[1] During pregnancy, it is important for families and their social support systems to be aware of signs and symptoms of new or worsening mental health challenges, and where to turn for help. It is also important to keep in mind that many people may feel stigma around mental health and its treatment – making it all the more important to provide compassionate, culturally sensitive support.

Some community and social service providers have mental health training, but many do not. Even when they do, it may not be within the scope of their current role to provide clinical intervention. In these circumstances, programs have often found it critical to have a professional mental health consultant who can provide guidance and support for staff whose clients are experiencing mental health challenges. This could be a mental health professional who works in your organization, or an external consultant who comes in on an as-needed basis. Yet even if you are not a mental health professional, you and your fellow community and social service providers can still play a critical role in supporting the mental health of your pregnant and postpartum clients.

This chapter focuses on preventing, identifying, and responding to mental health needs during and after pregnancy, including a discussion of research on this topic, practice

DOI: 10.4324/9781003476474-3

implications for your work, and reflections on your role as community and social service providers. Throughout this chapter, you will also hear the stories of Emily Cook Dyches, a loving mother who lost her life following serious postpartum mental health challenges, and the Wyoming Citizen Review Panel (WYCRP), which has worked hard to enhance its PAT home visiting services to better address the mental health needs of parents during and after pregnancy.

Research Summary and Implications for Community and Social Service Providers

Common Emotional Changes During Pregnancy and the Postpartum Period

Navigating pregnancy and the postpartum period is challenging for many families. For first-time parents, having a baby is a monumental life change. Balancing daily life, relationships, and/or employment with caring for a newborn is challenging, especially when coupled with hormonal and bodily changes. The transition into parenthood is sometimes referred to as *matrescence* (drawn from the word "maternal" or "mother"). What happens during matrescence is, in many ways, similar to what happens to young people during adolescence, in that the brain and body change to prepare for a new stage of life.[2] Those in matrescence go through a reorientation period during which they experience physical, psychological, and social changes – many of which are normal, but challenging (see Table 3.1 for examples).[3]

Before or after giving birth, whether it is their first or a subsequent birth, some experience short-term "baby blues," which can include symptoms such as stress, low mood and/or heightened emotions, and trouble concentrating (see Table 3.1).[4,5] Heightened anxiety is also common, especially in today's world with the overwhelming amount of parenting and health-related information available through the internet.

It can be challenging to identify whether mental health challenges in pregnancy and the early postpartum period are baby blues or mild anxiety, versus potentially more serious mental health concerns such as clinical depression or anxiety. Understanding an individual's context can assist community and social service providers to identify those who may be at risk for clinical mental health diagnoses, while also supporting all individuals with preventive mental health education and awareness.[6]

Table 3.1 Common Mental Health Changes and Clinical Warning Signs During Pregnancy and the Postpartum Period[113]

Examples of Common Changes in Mood and Related Areas	*Warning Signs and Symptoms of Clinical Depression*	*Examples of Common Worries and Behaviors*	*Warning Signs and Symptoms of Clinical Anxiety*
Mild, temporary mood fluctuations (i.e., irritability, overwhelm, sadness)	Feeling down, hopeless, moody, or angry for two weeks or longer	Feeling nervous about pregnancy or childbirth	Extreme or debilitating fear of pregnancy or childbirth
Occasional self-doubt or fluctuations in confidence (i.e., "Am I doing a good job?")	Feeling ashamed, guilty, or worthless for two weeks or longer	Mild anxiety about the life changes and stressors that come with pregnancy, postpartum, and early parenthood	Worrying constantly and excessively about many things; racing thoughts

(*Continued*)

Table 3.1 (Continued)

Examples of Common Changes in Mood and Related Areas	*Warning Signs and Symptoms of Clinical Depression*	*Examples of Common Worries and Behaviors*	*Warning Signs and Symptoms of Clinical Anxiety*
Mixed emotions about one's changing body, identity, and role	Severe self-esteem difficulties and/or difficulties coping with changes for two weeks or longer	Mild, temporary mood fluctuations (i.e., irritability, overwhelm)	Feeling irritable or angry much of the time
Gradual changes in social relationships	Withdrawing from friends and family for two weeks or longer	Occasional physical symptoms of anxiety in stress-provoking situations (i.e., increased heart rate)	Frequent or severe symptoms of physical anxiety (i.e., nausea, hyperventilating, panic attacks)
Gradual changes in daily activities or hobbies	Loss of interest in usual activities or hobbies, and/or struggling to feel pleasure or joy for two or more weeks	Trying to figure out plans and routines for navigating pregnancy, postpartum, and early parenthood, and feeling frustrated when things do not go as planned	Significant rigidity around plans and routines (i.e., sleep, feeding) and struggling to cope when things do not go as planned
Intermittent tearfulness	Frequent or uncontrollable crying Thoughts of harming oneself or the baby	Mild anxiety about the health and well-being of oneself and the baby	Excessively worrying that harm will come to oneself or the baby, and as a result being unable to sleep, to leave the baby briefly with another trusted adult, and/or go out in public with the baby

Putting It Into Practice

- ***Support parents in exploring and developing their parenting identity.*** Provide pregnant and postpartum clients with psychoeducation about matrescence, the phenomenon of becoming a parent, as described earlier in this chapter, along with opportunities to reflect on this evolution. You can also provide reassurance that one's identity as a parent does not emerge overnight and normalize the range of feelings that can accompany this transitional time.

Take Time to Reflect

Review the list of common mental health challenges and clinical warning signs during pregnancy and the postpartum period (Table 3.1). If you have ever been pregnant, reflect on whether you experienced anything listed. If you have never been pregnant, think about someone you know. What helped you or the other person to cope with the ups and downs of pregnancy and/or the postpartum period? How did you assess the seriousness of the symptoms or warning signs?

Emily's Story ∞

Emily Cook Dyches' husband Eric publicly remembers her as "a committed mother, a caring daughter, a loving sister, a compassionate and kind neighbor and, most importantly . . . the beautiful and supportive girl of my dreams."[7] They had four children together and decided to add a fifth to their loving fold. Shortly after giving birth, Emily experienced complications and nearly died. She was medically cleared for discharge from the hospital two days later; however, emotionally, she struggled with significant anxiety and fear after this traumatic event, in addition to the ups and downs of the postpartum period, including adjusting to life as a mother of five and breastfeeding difficulties. With her husband's support, she sought help and was diagnosed with and engaged in treatment for postpartum depression and anxiety, though it was often challenging to navigate the mental healthcare system. A few weeks before her youngest child's first birthday, Emily experienced a severe panic attack while riding in a moving vehicle. In a state of overwhelm, she exited the vehicle and tragically lost her life. Today, Eric has founded The Emily Effect, an organization that provides support and resources to individuals and families struggling with mood disorders during and after pregnancy. Their mission "is to raise awareness through light, hope, and knowledge . . . in her name."[7]

Depression

Depression is a serious condition that affects millions worldwide before, during, and after pregnancy. Depression includes a wide range of emotional, cognitive, and physical symptoms (see Table 3.1). It is both a cause and effect of maternal and infant health problems.[8] Depression during the prenatal and postpartum stages can also be experienced by parents who did not give birth. It can also have negative impacts on bonding between parents and their babies and is associated with increased risk of self-harm and suicide.[9,10] Depression is also one of the most treatable mental health conditions, especially when it is detected early – making it a very important condition for community and social service providers to know about.

Rates of Depression

Research has found that rates of depression (which were already concerningly high) have grown in recent years during pregnancy and the postpartum period. For example, a large study in the United States found that the number of individuals who gave birth in hospitals and were diagnosed with depression increased seven-fold – from 4.1 diagnoses out of 1,000 people in the year 2000, to 28.7 diagnoses out of 1,000 people in the year 2015.[11] Several recent studies have found that approximately one-quarter of pregnant and postpartum individuals meet diagnostic criteria for depression,[12,13] though some studies with populations with high levels of stressors or risk factors have reported rates of 50% or more.[14]

Research suggests that some groups are at increased risk for developing depression during pregnancy and the postpartum period. For example, some studies have found that people of color in the United States may be more likely to experience depression symptoms than White people,[11,12,15,16,17] though White people may be more likely to receive formal diagnoses. Heightened rates of depression have also been found among those with public versus private insurance.[11] These patterns are likely related to systemic inequities in stressors, access to mental healthcare, and more. See the following "*Risk and Protective Factors*" section for further discussion.

Timing of Depression

Although people commonly think of postpartum depression, it is important to know that depression can emerge at any point during pregnancy or the postpartum period. Depression during pregnancy has been linked to increased risk of ongoing depression during the postpartum period.[18,19] After giving birth, many individuals experience a brief period of mood fluctuation known as the "baby blues" (see Table 3.1). When symptoms are more severe and last two weeks or more, the possibility of postpartum depression should be considered.

Postpartum depression does not always emerge right away. In fact, one study of young mothers found that among those who screened positive for depression, 15% screened positive for the first time between six and 12 months postpartum and that the most common time to screen positive (23%) was at 12 months postpartum.[20] These findings highlight the importance of screening for depression symptoms throughout pregnancy and the entire first year postpartum.

Risk and Protective Factors

Many risk and protective factors for depression during and after pregnancy have been identified. Numerous studies have found that those with histories of pre-pregnancy mental health challenges (i.e., depression, anxiety, substance use, trauma) are at increased risk of experiencing depression after getting pregnant.[18,21,22,23,24,25,26,27,28] Pregnancy planning has also been linked to risk of depression. Research has found that anywhere between one-third and three-fourths of pregnancies were unplanned, and that those with unanticipated pregnancies are significantly more likely to experience depression and psychological distress during pregnancy and beyond.[21,29,30,31]

Individuals with significant life stressors (i.e., material hardship or poverty, food insecurity, intimate partner violence, community violence, racial stress) are also at increased risk for experiencing depression during and after pregnancy, especially if those stressors are severe and/or multiple in nature.[12,14,15,21,32,33,34,35,36,37,38,39,40,41,42,43] Pregnancy- and delivery-related stressors (i.e., knowledge about pregnancy, pregnancy complications, unexpected C-section delivery, birth trauma, severe infant illness) have also been linked to increased risk for depression.[44,45,46,47,48] Alternatively, high levels of social support and socio-cultural connections have been shown to be protective against depression during pregnancy and the postpartum period.[49,50,51,52,53,54,55]

Take Action

What protocols does your organization currently have in place for screening pregnant and postpartum clients for depression? If there are not protocols in place, consider who you can speak to about this. If there are protocols in place, consider how frequently screenings take place during pregnancy and the postpartum period. As the research described above suggests, it is important to screen throughout these entire time periods through at least one year postpartum.

Anxiety Disorders

Like depression, anxiety disorders affect a significant proportion of individuals before, during, and after pregnancy; however, they are often overlooked by both providers and clients.[56] Anxiety disorders encompass a wide range of emotional, cognitive, and physical symptoms (see Table 3.1), and can be both causes and effects of physical health problems. Anxiety disorders can also have negative affects on bonding with the baby. The good news is that anxiety disorders are highly treatable – making this another important condition for community and social service providers to know about.

Rates of Anxiety Disorders

The estimated prevalence of anxiety disorders during pregnancy and postpartum ranges across sources and studies.[57] However, rates of 15–20% have commonly been found.[58,59] Some research has suggested that, in the United States, rates of anxiety may be particularly high among Black mothers due to the stressors that this group faces.[60] Other research has found that Black mothers and other mothers of color may be less likely to be diagnosed with anxiety disorders than their White counterparts (even if they meet diagnostic criteria), likely due to disparities in healthcare access and culturally sensitive screening.[61]

Timing of Anxiety Disorders

Evidence suggests that individuals may be screened less often for anxiety than depression during pregnancy and the postpartum period.[56] A large study found that the best time for screening and identifying anxiety disorders was in early pregnancy.[62] Similarly, in a study of pregnant and postpartum Latinas, researchers found that overall rates of positive anxiety screenings were highest in the first trimester of pregnancy, with some differences in whether those symptoms persisted or decreased over time based on race and ethnicity.[63]

Risk and Protective Factors

Individuals with previous histories of anxiety disorders or other mental health challenges are at increased risk for developing anxiety disorders during and after pregnancy.[57,64] Having an unanticipated pregnancy has also been identified as a significant risk factor for anxiety.[29] This finding may provide context for why some experience heightened anxiety in the first trimester of pregnancy. Research has also found that certain groups are more likely to report high levels of anxiety symptoms during pregnancy, including those with low incomes or material hardship, those who live in areas with high levels of segregation, and those who are in relationships with unsupportive partners.[32,57,60] Having a previous difficult or traumatic delivery experience has also been linked to increased risk.[44,64] Alternatively, as with depression, high levels of social support and socio-cultural connections have been shown to be protective against anxiety during pregnancy.[50,54]

Putting It Into Practice

- ***Encourage social support, especially during the postpartum period.*** Those who stay connected to their loved ones during the postpartum period are more likely to maintain good mental health, whereas those whose social connections decrease during this time are more likely to experience depression. Interestingly, some research has suggested that joining new social groups during the postpartum period does not have a major impact on depression symptoms.[65] It makes sense that, particularly for new parents who are already struggling with depression, the idea of meeting new people may be overwhelming – and for many new parents (whether their mental health is relatively good or they are struggling), it can even be difficult to find the time or energy to connect with family and long-time friends. Here, community and social service providers can make a positive difference by validating the importance of maintaining connections with trusted loved ones during the postpartum period. When framed as an important strategy for promoting the parent's well-being (and thus, the baby's), parents may be more likely to buy in.

- ***Provide universal education about depression and anxiety during and after pregnancy.*** It is important to provide all pregnant and postpartum clients with information about mental health, including (but not limited to) potential warning signs of more serious mental health problems such as depression or anxiety disorders. Informing clients that these problems affect many people can reduce the stigma around mental health, and make clients feel more comfortable opening up about any challenges they have been experiencing.

Other Mental Health Conditions

Depression and anxiety disorders are the most common mental health conditions during and after pregnancy, however, there are several other conditions (i.e., mania, psychosis, obsessive-compulsive disorder, post-traumatic stress) that, while rare, can be quite serious. It is important for community and social service providers to have some awareness of these conditions so that they can appropriately support and refer their clients. Table 3.2 outlines examples of potential warning signs to look for.

Table 3.2 Example Warning Signs of Other Potentially Serious Prenatal and Postpartum Mental Health Difficulties

Thoughts	*Feelings*	*Behavior*
• Hallucinations (seeing, hearing, smelling, tasting, or feelings things that other people cannot perceive) • Delusions or paranoia (unusual thoughts, fears, beliefs, or suspicions that are probably untrue) • Flashbacks or frequent, intense nightmares, particularly around traumatic experiences • Frequent, unwanted, distressing thoughts or mental images about harming the baby	• Unusually high, irritable, or agitated mood • Feeling disconnected from one's body • Feeling disconnected from the baby	• Significantly increased or decreased activity levels • Increased risk-taking behavior • Not feeling the need to sleep • Bizarre, confused, or disorganized behavior or speech • Rituals or compulsions (i.e., checking, cleaning, counting) • Severe difficulties with self-care or hygiene • Avoiding and/or being afraid to be left alone with the baby

Self-Care Moment

The next section discusses suicide during and after pregnancy. Take reading breaks as needed to take care of yourself.

Suicidality

Suicidality (the risk of suicide, or killing oneself) is a serious symptom that can go hand in hand with depression, anxiety disorders, and other mental health conditions during pregnancy and the postpartum period. There is a common perception that the joy and increased responsibility of becoming a parent may be protective against suicide; however, research suggests that the risk of suicidality actually increases during pregnancy and the postpartum period, due to accompanying stressors and biological changes.[66] Therefore, it is essential that community and social service providers know about the warning signs of suicidality so that they can help their clients get the help needed to maintain safety.

Rates of Suicidality

A small but significant proportion of individuals experience suicidal thoughts or urges to engage in self-harm during or after pregnancy. One large review study found that the estimated proportion of pregnant women who experience suicidal thoughts could be as high as 33%; other studies have offered lower estimates.[67,68,69] Other work has found that in the United States, the prevalence of suicidal thoughts during pregnancy more than doubled in the mid-2000s.[70] Other work from the same time period has similarly found significant increases in intentional self-harm among this group.[70] Research suggests that rates of suicidal thoughts may be higher among mothers of color and those with low incomes.[70,71]

Research suggests that only a small percentage of pregnant and postpartum individuals who experience suicidal thoughts have the intention, plans, and means to end their lives. However, it is important to emphasize that all suicidal thoughts should be taken seriously and that risk evaluations should only be conducted by qualified mental health professionals.[68] In the United States, it has been estimated that approximately 2–5 completed suicides occur among every 100,000 individuals who give birth to a live infant.[72]

Timing of Suicidality

Suicide can occur at any point during or after pregnancy; however, research suggests that it is most likely to occur well into the postpartum period. For example, a large study in California found that pregnancy-related suicides were most likely to occur between six and 12 months postpartum.[73] Similarly, another study reported that 62% of pregnancy-related suicides occurred between 43 days and one year postpartum, 24% occurred during pregnancy, and 14% occurred 42 days or less after giving birth.[74]

Risk and Protective Factors

In addition to current depression, research suggests that those with a pre-pregnancy history of depression or other mental health conditions are significantly more likely to experience suicidal thoughts during or after pregnancy[67,75] Individuals who feel like they are a burden to others are at increased risk for suicidal behavior, as are those who perceive that their mental health challenges are not being sufficiently treated or supported.[76,77] Low social support, C-section delivery, and other complications or injuries during labor and delivery have also been identified as risk factors.[63]

Unfortunately, research on protective factors against self-harm and suicide during and after pregnancy has been relatively limited. Broader research around suicidality has found that social support is an important protective factor for individuals experiencing suicidal thoughts.[78] Timely identification and access to effective, culturally sensitive mental healthcare is also undoubtedly important.

Putting It Into Practice

- ***Know signs of potential suicidality and other urgent mental health symptoms.*** Suicidality and severe mental illness are relatively rare during pregnancy and the postpartum period. However, when they do occur, quick and careful action is needed to ensure safety. It is therefore essential that all community and social service providers know the warning signs of potential suicidality and other urgent mental health symptoms (see Table 3.2 for a list of examples). Sometimes, these signs and symptoms may come up during a mental health screening; other times, the provider may simply notice them while observing or talking with a pregnant or postpartum client. These concerns can emerge at any point during and after pregnancy, though as noted earlier in this chapter, suicidality is often highest well into the postpartum period.

  It is also important that community and social service providers know their organization's protocol for responding to potential suicidality or other urgent mental health symptoms. If a protocol does not already exist, one should be developed in coordination with a professional mental health consultant. The protocol should include a list of local resources (i.e., local/national emergency numbers, local/national suicide and crisis lifelines, local emergency departments where clients can be evaluated.)

Take Action

Take a few minutes to update your knowledge of local suicide prevention resources. Open an online search engine and type "[name of your country or town] suicide prevention." The results will likely include suicide prevention organizations, national suicide and crisis lifelines, and more. Take some time to peruse these websites, taking note of any handouts or resources that might be helpful to share with your colleagues or clients.

Screening and Intervention

The Wyoming Citizen Review Panel (WYCRP): Bringing Hope During and After Pregnancy Δ

After noticing a high number of parents and caregivers struggling with depression, the WYCRP affiliate of PAT began offering depression screenings and treatment referrals to parents enrolled in home visiting services. In doing so, WYCRP noticed several barriers that seemed to prevent caregivers from accessing the services to which they were referred: services were not readily available, parents were put on a waitlist, parents lacked the childcare and transportation required to receive services, unreliable internet service prevented virtual assistance, and there was an underlying stigma associated with accessing mental health treatment.

WYCRP thought long and hard about potential solutions to these challenges and barriers. Ultimately, they found Mothers and Babies, an evidence-based intervention to help pregnant families and new parents manage stress and prevent postpartum depression. In 2021, WYCRP staff were trained in the Mothers and Babies curriculum and began to incorporate it into their home visiting services. Within six months, the percentage of primary parents and caregivers that initiated mental health services following a positive mental health screening more than tripled, and by the following year, WYCRP had 36 families participating in Mothers and Babies with a total of 113 sessions completed.

The WYCRP program found that Mothers and Babies can have a positive impact on the mental health of families and their home visitors. In completing the program, many families reported positive feedback, additional opportunities for reflection, and increased openness to accessing outside mental health services. One mother was empowered to reach out to a support person instead of giving up during a crisis, and she got the help she needed to overcome the situation. Several home visitors shared that they personally completed the Mothers and Babies activities and found them immensely valuable in their own personal lives.

Through the integration of Mothers and Babies into home visiting services, WYCRP has been able to address the mental health needs of more families, especially those in rural or low-resource areas. This approach helps to promote positive health outcomes during and after pregnancy, establish more trusting and communicative relationships, and work toward the destigmatization of mental health concerns and treatment options.

For more information on the WYCRP PAT program and its integration of the Mothers and Babies curriculum, visit <https://wypat.org>.

Given the prevalence of mental health challenges during and after pregnancy, there is a critical need for effective screening and intervention strategies in both healthcare and broader community settings (including home visiting). Unfortunately, many individuals do not receive mental health screenings until late in pregnancy, resulting in delayed identification and treatment of conditions. In addition, some groups are less likely than others to be screened at all (for example, publicly insured people and those without pre-pregnancy histories of mental health challenges).[79,80,81] Research has identified several promising strategies which may help to address this gap, including conducting in-home screenings, incorporating technology, and having established referral processes in place for other services if a screening identifies an issue.

Identification and Screening

It can be difficult to distinguish between normal fluctuations in mental health during and after pregnancy, and more serious conditions like depression or anxiety disorders.[82] To address this, providers (both medical providers and community and social service providers) can use standardized screening or assessment tools like the Edinburgh Postnatal Depression Scale and the Patient Health Questionnaire that ask people about their mood, level of anxiety and insomnia, and other health concerns during pregnancy and the postpartum period. In addition to asking these questions, it is important the providers create environments in which clients feel safe opening about any struggles they are facing. One study found that 1 in 5 postpartum women did not disclose their depressive symptoms to their provider, and that those who had high levels of stress and low levels of social support were less likely to disclose.[83]

Innovative Screening Strategies

In recent years, several innovative strategies have been developed for conducting mental health screenings during pregnancy and the postpartum period. For example, one study investigated the feasibility of a text-based screening program for postpartum mental health.[84] For the first 12 weeks after giving birth, participants received a two-question depression screening every two weeks, along with multiple text messages a week about postpartum mental health topics. Ninety-nine percent of participants responded to at least one of the text screenings, and about two-thirds responded to all six screenings. Those who screened positive were offered an appointment with a mental healthcare provider; approximately half of these individuals ultimately attended the appointment. Among those who completed a satisfaction survey, over three-quarters recommended that text-based depression screenings be offered to all individuals during the postpartum period.

Another study reported on the process of developing a postpartum toolkit (screening questionnaire, feedback template, and decision aid) for mothers addressing their behavioral and psychosocial health during the postpartum period.[85] Pilot participants from diverse backgrounds reported that the toolkit was useful and easy to understand, and that they were likely to follow through on the goals that they had set for themselves using the toolkit.

Putting It Into Practice

- ***Conduct universal screenings for depression and anxiety.*** As noted earlier in this chapter, research has found that many individuals do not feel comfortable discussing sensitive topics with their healthcare providers during pregnancy and the postpartum period. Mental health screening within the context of a trusting, ongoing relationship with a community or social service provider can help to address this gap.

  Follow clear guidelines from reputable sources about when to screen pregnant and postpartum clients. While many existing guidelines were originally developed for healthcare providers, they can also be relevant and helpful for community and social service providers. For example, the Policy Center for Maternal Mental Health recommends conducting mental health screenings with all clients at least once during pregnancy (ideally late in the first trimester or early in the second trimester), at least once six weeks after birth, and at least one more time during the first year after birth.[86] As noted earlier in this chapter, some research has found that rates of positive screens for depression are highest at the end of the postpartum period (12 months after giving birth).

Several validated mental health screening tools are available for free public use. The American College of Obstetricians and Gynecologists and other organizations often maintain updated lists of tools on their websites.[87] Many of these measures can be used by community and social service providers without formal mental health training. However, it is still a good idea for organizations to train their staff in how to use these measures with their specific client population, and to work with a mental health consultant to develop protocols for how to appropriately handle positive screens (i.e., providing referrals, obtaining mental health crisis services).

It is important to keep in mind that anyone can experience depression, anxiety, or other mental health conditions, and thus to conduct preventive screenings with all pregnant and postpartum clients. However, it may be especially important to conduct screenings with clients who had previous histories of depression, anxiety, or other mental health conditions before they got pregnant, since research has shown that this group is at particularly high risk for mental health challenges during pregnancy and the postpartum period.

There is also growing recognition of the importance of conducting depression screenings with partners or co-parents, who often are also experiencing major life changes. Approaching mental health and wellness through a whole-family lens during and after pregnancy can influence the family's overall well-being as family members navigate the transition to parenthood or expand their family.

Clinical Mental Health Treatment

Many clinical mental health treatments (i.e., psychotherapy, medication) have been shown to be effective in addressing mental health concerns during and after pregnancy. However, research indicates that many mental health needs go unmet during these periods. For example, several large studies in the United States have reported that less than half of those who experience clinical mental health conditions during pregnancy receive any treatment, with some studies reporting treatment rates as low as 12%.[32,88,89,90,91] Research finds that people of color often access mental health treatment at lower rates than White people.[90,92,93] Commonly reported barriers to treatment include financial concerns, logistical issues (i.e., transportation, time off work, childcare), personal and cultural understandings and beliefs around mental health and its treatment, and stigma.[13,67,90,91,94,95,96,97,98,99,100]

One study in the Midwest United States reported that during the postpartum stage, women who felt overwhelmed and under-supported in their life overall (not just around childcare responsibilities) were more likely to seek help for postpartum depression. Research has also suggested that individuals with ongoing medical issues, tobacco use, or histories of experiencing abuse may be more likely to utilize mental health services, perhaps because they are already involved in the healthcare system and more likely to be screened.[90] Embedding care in other settings (i.e., adult or pediatric primary care, community centers), as well as offering in-home or telehealth services, have also been linked to increased participation in treatment, particularly for those with low incomes.[94,101,102]

Putting It Into Practice

- ***Facilitate access to mental health services.*** After identifying possible mental health concerns, the next step is to connect the affected individual to mental health services. This is not always easy. Many communities have limited mental health services, or the services that do exist have long waitlists or are not a good fit. Sometimes, people may be reluctant to engage in services. A good first step can be for the individual to speak with their healthcare provider (if they have one) about their mental health symptoms, and/or by contacting their insurance company (if they have insurance) to learn more about their healthcare options. In recent years, the rise of telehealth has offered new avenues for people to access mental healthcare. You can make a difference by talking to clients about their thoughts, feelings, and potential concerns about mental healthcare, and by providing them with a list of trusted providers and resources. You can also help clients to problem-solve around factors that might make it hard for them to obtain care, such as financial barriers, transportation challenges, or childcare coverage.

  At the organizational level, strategic collaborations with healthcare providers and other social service providers can be very beneficial for facilitating families' access to services. When possible, written agreements that specify coordination of efforts can increase families' opportunities for timely access.
  Stay up to date about primary contacts and current processes at community agencies that can be shared with families to maximize their success in obtaining needed resources or services. Networking with representatives of other organizations, participating in professional associations, and being a part of community collaborations all help professionals stay up to date about viable options for mental health services and avenues to optimize access to these services.

Take Action

If you are not already familiar with them, investigate what kinds of strategic collaborations your organization has in place with local mental health providers and agencies. Confirm whether your organization has a method for maintaining up-to-date contact information, referral protocols, and other details.

Other Support Strategies

While individual therapy and medication have been the traditional treatment plans for perinatal depression, recent research has been looking into the effectiveness of other forms of treatment. Many of these treatments fall into the category of group programs. Some examples include the following.

- Mothers and Babies (MB): A perinatal depression prevention intervention that can be offered in 1:1 or group formats (www.mothersandbabiesprogram.org/);
- Family Foundations (FF): A transition to parenthood program for couples (www.cebc4cw.org/program/family-foundations/detailed); and
- Postpartum support groups.

These programs have received positive feedback from participants about enjoying the content and format of the interventions and reporting that they felt supported and more likely to share symptoms with their fellow group members.[103] However, some challenges to group programs include issues around attendance, transportation, and implementation.[104]

There have also been significant developments in strategies for community engagement in program planning. Two prime examples include the New Haven Mental Health Outreach for Mothers (MOMS) Partnership and the Massachusetts Child Psychiatry Access Project (MCPAP) for Moms. MOMS is a community-academic partnership that developed a model for training community health workers in maternal mental health using 12 primary content areas. Program evaluation has revealed significant pre-post changes in participants' attitudes, perceived self-efficacy, and control following training.[105] Meanwhile, MCPAP is a population-based program that helps providers address perinatal depression. MCPAP includes trainings and toolkits on depression screening, assessment, and treatment; telephonic access to perinatal psychiatric consultation for providers; and care coordination to link women with individual psychotherapy and support groups. Program evaluation has revealed that, in its first 18 months, MCPAP served 1,123 women at a cost of only $0.70 per woman per month.[106]

Mental Health Among Fathers and Other Co-Parents

While this book and chapter primarily focus on the experiences of the parent who is pregnant, it is important to acknowledge that fathers and other co-parents also experience significant life changes during pregnancy and the postpartum period, which can contribute to mental health challenges similar to those previously described.[107] For example, recent research has estimated that 8–10% of fathers experience postpartum depression, related to many of the same personal and social risk factors described earlier in this chapter.[108] When the mental health challenges of fathers and co-parents are left untreated, they can negatively affect bonding with the baby, as well as the mental health and well-being of their partners.[109,110,111]

Research has shown that many fathers and co-parents under-report their mental health symptoms or do not realize that the thoughts and emotions they are experiencing are clinically significant.[112] Using standardized mental health screening tools has been found helpful for more accurately identifying fathers and co-parents who are struggling with their mental health.[112] Similar to what was described earlier in this chapter, fathers and co-parents also commonly struggle to access effective, culturally sensitive mental health services – underscoring the important role that community and social service providers can play in providing education, encouragement, and referrals.

Putting It Into Practice

- ***Approach the topic of mental health from a whole-family lens.*** Ask fathers and other co-parents how they are coping with the pregnancy and/or postpartum period. Consider conducting universal screenings for depression and anxiety during pregnancy and after childbirth with fathers and other co-parents. Ensure that you have resources and referrals ready that are tailored to the needs of fathers and other co-parents.

Your Role as a Community or Social Service Provider

Listening and Learning

The data and information in this chapter present a picture of the mental health challenges that can occur during pregnancy and the postpartum period. Understanding the data, statistics, and stories specific to your community will help you to tailor your services to the issues, needs, and strengths of your local community and the families within it. Consider: what do you already know about the prenatal and postpartum mental health challenges that occur in your local community (for example, how often they occur and which types of challenges are most common)? How can you learn more (i.e., researching information and local data, listening to personal stories of different kinds of families in your community)?

In addition to researching local data and statistics, you can also make a difference by closely attending to the sometimes-subtle changes that signal that someone may be struggling with their mental health. Utilize organizational resources such as consultation or reflective supervision with a mental health professional to process your observations, determine how to bring them back to the client, and help them take steps toward obtaining mental health supports or services.

Advocating

Availability and accessibility of mental health services can vary significantly in different communities, and for different individuals within the same community. Consider: what you know about the quality and accessibility of mental health services in your community? How have you served as a bridge between those you work with and mental health resources? How do you stay up to date with contact information, referral protocols, and other details for local mental health services?

As discussed earlier in this book, your role as a community or service provider operates on two levels: (a) your individual work with families; and (b) your work with systems, including local mental healthcare. The lessons outlined in this chapter pertain to both levels of work and also point to the need for broader advocacy around mental health for pregnant and postpartum people. You can advocate within your organization – for example, for the development or refinement of mental health screening protocols, for an ongoing relationship with a mental health consultant, for increasing professional development around mental health for staff, or for embedding additional mental health support strategies or interventions into your work with clients. You can also advocate outside of your organization in the community at large by lifting up policies, programs, and initiatives that will support mental health and well-being during and after pregnancy.

Take Time to Reflect

Reflecting on the practice implications throughout this chapter and your role as a community or social service provider, what is one area where you believe you are already doing an excellent job? What is one area where you could improve your professional practice or deepen your understanding and knowledge?

Take Action

Now that you have reflected on an area where you could improve your professional practice, create a SMART goal to make it happen, described as follows.

- **S**pecific
- **M**easurable
- **A**chievable
- **R**elevant
- **T**ime-Bound

For example, imagine that you would like to increase mental health screenings with your postpartum clients. A SMART goal might be:

> Postpartum depression is a condition that affects a lot of people, including some of my clients (**Relevant**). By the end of this quarter (**Time-Bound**), I will intentionally increase my use of the Patient Health Questionnaire-9 depression screening measure, so that I complete at least one screening with at least 50% of my postpartum caseload (**Measurable, Specific, Achievable**). I will track my progress and screenings in my caseload spreadsheet and client records.

Key Takeaways From This Chapter

1. Depression and anxiety disorders are among the most common mental health challenges during pregnancy and the postpartum period. These conditions can affect anyone at any point during or after pregnancy, and can also affect fathers and other co-parents. They are also very treatable with medication and/or therapy, especially when identified early.
2. Some groups are more likely to experience mental health challenges during and after pregnancy (i.e., those with pre-pregnancy mental health histories, those with high levels of stressors, those who experience other complications during pregnancy or childbirth, those with low levels of social support). This is largely due to barriers in access to high-quality mental healthcare, as well as other SDOH.
3. Community and social service providers can take many steps to promote the mental health of pregnant and postpartum families, even if they are not mental health professionals. The strong relationships that they build with families over time put them in a strong position to make a difference.

References

1. Logue, T. C., Wen, T., Monk, C., Guglielminotti, J., Huang, Y., Wright, J. D., D'Alton, M. E., & Friedman, A. M. (2022). Trends in and complications associated with mental health condition diagnoses during delivery hospitalizations. *American Journal of Obstetrics and Gynecology*, *226*(3), 405.e1–405.e16. https://doi.org/10.1016/j.ajog.2021.09.021
2. Orchard, E. R., Rutherford, H. J. V., Holmes, A. J., & Jamadar, S. D. (2023). Matrescence: Lifetime impact of motherhood on cognition and the brain. *Trends in Cognitive Sciences*, *27*(3), 302–316. https://doi.org/10.1016/j.tics.2022.12.002
3. Raphael, D. (Ed.). (1975). Matrescence, becoming a mother, a "new/old" rite de passage. In *Being female: Reproduction, power, and change* (pp. 65–71). Mouton. https://doi.org/10.1515/9783110813128.65
4. Banasiewicz, J., Zaręba, K., Bińkowska, M., Rozenek, H., Wójtowicz, S., & Jakiel, G. (2020). Perinatal predictors of postpartum depression: Results of a retrospective comparative study. *Journal of Clinical Medicine*, *9*(9), 2952. https://doi.org/10.3390/jcm9092952
5. Dhaliwal, S. K., Dabelea, D., Lee-Winn, A. E., Glueck, D. H., Wilkening, G., & Perng, W. (2022). Characterization of maternal psychosocial stress during pregnancy: The Healthy Start Study. *Women's Health Reports*, *3*(1), 698–708. https://doi.org/10.1089/whr.2022.0011
6. Robinson, M., Pennell, C. E., McLean, N. J., Tearne, J. E., Oddy, W. H., & Newnham, J. P. (2015). Risk perception in pregnancy: Context, consequences, and clinical implications. *European Psychologist*, *20*(2), 120–127. https://doi.org/10.1027/1016-9040/a000212
7. *Who was Emily Cook Dyches?* https://theemilyeffect.org/emilys-story/
8. Miller, E. S., Saade, G. R., Simhan, H. N., Monk, C., Haas, D. M., Silver, R. M., Mercer, B. M., Parry, S., Wing, D. A., Reddy, U. M., & Grobman, W. A. (2022). Trajectories of antenatal depression and adverse pregnancy outcomes. *American Journal of Obstetrics and Gynecology*, *226*(1), 108.e1–108.e9. https://doi.org/10.1016/j.ajog.2021.07.007
9. Hildingsson, I., & Rubertsson, C. (2022). Postpartum bonding and association with depressive symptoms and prenatal attachment in women with fear of birth. *BMC Pregnancy and Childbirth*, *22*(1), 66. https://doi.org/10.1186/s12884-021-04367-3
10. Saharoy, R., Potdukhe, A., Wanjari, M., & Taksande, A. B. (2023). Postpartum depression and maternal care: Exploring the complex effects on mothers and infants. *Cureus*, *15*(7), e41381. https://doi.org/10.7759/cureus.41381
11. Haight, S. C., Byatt, N., Simas, T. A. M., Robbins, C. L., & Ko, J. Y. (2019). Recorded diagnoses of depression during United States delivery hospitalizations, 2000–2015. *Obstetrics and Gynecology*, *133*(6), 1216. https://doi.org/10.1097/AOG.0000000000003291
12. Benatar, S., Cross-Barnet, C., Johnston, E., & Hill, I. (2020). Prenatal depression: Assessment and outcomes among Medicaid participants. *The Journal of Behavioral Health Services & Research*, *47*(3), 409–423. https://doi.org/10.1007/s11414-020-09689-2
13. Corrigan, C. P., Kwasky, A. N., & Groh, C. J. (2015). Social support, postpartum depression, and professional assistance: A survey of mothers in the Midwestern United States. *The Journal of Perinatal Education*, *24*(1), 48–60. https://doi.org/10.1891/1058-1243.24.1.48
14. Buzi, R. S., Smith, P. B., Kozinetz, C. A., Peskin, M. F., & Wiemann, C. M. (2015). A socioecological framework to assessing depression among pregnant teens. *Maternal and Child Health Journal*, *19*(10), 2187–2194. https://doi.org/10.1007/s10995-015-1733-y
15. Mukherjee, S., Fennie, K., Coxe, S., Madhivanan, P., & Trepka, M. J. (2018). Racial and ethnic differences in the relationship between antenatal stressful life events and postpartum depression among women in the United States: Does provider communication on perinatal depression minimize the risk? *Ethnicity & Health*, *23*(5), 542–565. https://doi.org/10.1080/13557858.2017.1280137
16. Shorter, J. M., Koelper, N., Sonalkar, S., Oquendo, M. A., Sammel, M. D., & Schreiber, C. A. (2021). Racial disparities in mental health outcomes among women with early pregnancy loss. *Obstetrics and Gynecology*, *137*(1), 156–163. https://doi.org/10.1097/AOG.0000000000004212
17. Shin, S. H., Ksinan Jiskrova, G., Kimbrough, T., Dina, K. T., Lee, E. O., & Ayers, C. E. (2021). Maternal adverse childhood experiences and postpartum depressive symptoms in young, low-income women. *Psychiatry Research*, *296*, 113679. https://doi.org/10.1016/j.psychres.2020.113679
18. McCall-Hosenfeld, J. S., Phiri, K., Schaefer, E., Zhu, J., & Kjerulff, K. (2016). Trajectories of depressive symptoms throughout the peri-and postpartum period: Results from the first

baby study. *Journal of Women's Health, 25*(11), 1112–1121. https://doi.org/10.1089/jwh.2015.5310

19. Wilcox, M., McGee, B. A., Ionescu, D. F., Leonte, M., LaCross, L., Reps, J., & Wildenhaus, K. (2021). Perinatal depressive symptoms often start in the prenatal rather than postpartum period: Results from a longitudinal study. *Archives of Women's Mental Health, 24*(1), 119–131. https://doi.org/10.1007/s00737-020-01017-z
20. McKean, M., Caughey, A. B., Yuracko McKean, M. A., Cabana, M. D., & Flaherman, V. J. (2018). Postpartum depression: When should health care providers identify those at risk? *Clinical Pediatrics, 57*(6), 689–693. https://doi.org/10.1177/0009922817733696
21. Gauthreaux, C., Negron, J., Castellanos, D., Ward-Peterson, M., Castro, G., de la Vega, P. R., & Acuña, J. M. (2017). The association between pregnancy intendedness and experiencing symptoms of postpartum depression among new mothers in the United States, 2009 to 2011: A secondary analysis of PRAMS data. *Medicine, 96*(6). https://doi.org/10.1097/MD.0000000000005851
22. Grekin, R., Brock, R. L., & O'Hara, M. W. (2017). The effects of trauma on perinatal depression: Examining trajectories of depression from pregnancy through 24 months postpartum in an at-risk population. *Journal of Affective Disorders, 218*, 269–276. https://doi.org/10.1016/j.jad.2017.04.051
23. Kinser, P. A., Thacker, L. R., Lapato, D., Wagner, S., Roberson-Nay, R., Jobe-Shields, L., Amstadler, A., & York, T. P. (2018). Depressive symptom prevalence and predictors in the first half of pregnancy. *Journal of Women's Health, 27*(3), 369–376. https://doi.org/10.1089/jwh.2017.6426
24. Ruyak, S. L., Flores-Montoya, A., & Boursaw, B. (2017). Antepartum services and symptoms of postpartum depression in at-risk women. *Journal of Obstetric, Gynecologic & Neonatal Nursing, 46*(5), 696–708. https://doi.org/10.1016/j.jogn.2017.07.006
25. Sampson, M., Duron, J. F., Mauldin, R. L., Kao, D., & Davidson, M. (2017). Postpartum depression, risk factors, and child's home environment among mothers in a home visiting program. *Journal of Child and Family Studies, 26*(10), 2772–2781. https://doi.org/10.1007/s10826-017-0783-8
26. Ding, X., Liang, M., Wang, H., Song, Q., Guo, X., Su, W., Li, N., Liu, H., Ma, S., Zhou, X., & Sun, Y. (2023). Prenatal stressful life events increase the prevalence of postpartum depression: Evidence from prospective cohort studies. *Journal of Psychiatric Research, 160*, 263–271. https://doi.org/10.1016/j.jpsychires.2023.02.036
27. Edwards, M. V., Campbell, H. K., Miller, C. R., Vazirabadi, G., Fisher, E. K., & Mathews, K. J. (2022). Positive depression screening at the first prenatal visit in a low-income primarily Black population. *Journal of Health Care for the Poor and Underserved, 33*(1), 20–32. https://doi.org/10.1353/hpu.2022.0004
28. Hernandez, N. D., Francis, S., Allen, M., Bellamy, E., Sims, O. T., Oh, H., Guillaume, D., Parker, A., & Chandler, R. (2022). Prevalence and predictors of symptoms of perinatal mood and anxiety disorders among a sample of urban Black women in the South. *Maternal and Child Health Journal, 26*(4), 770–777. https://doi.org/10.1007/s10995-022-03425-2
29. Gariepy, A. M., Lundsberg, L. S., Miller, D., Stanwood, N. L., & Yonkers, K. A. (2016). Are pregnancy planning and pregnancy timing associated with maternal psychiatric illness, psychological distress and support during pregnancy? *Journal of Affective Disorders, 205*, 87–94. https://doi.org/10.1016/j.jad.2016.06.058
30. Barber, G. A., & Steinberg, J. R. (2022). The association between pregnancy intention, fertility treatment use, and postpartum depression. *Social Science & Medicine (1982), 314*, 115439. https://doi.org/10.1016/j.socscimed.2022.115439
31. Sasaki, N., Ikeda, M., & Nishi, D. (2022). Long-term influence of unintended pregnancy on psychological distress: A large sample retrospective cross-sectional study. *Archives of Women's Mental Health, 25*(6), 1119–1127. https://doi.org/10.1007/s00737-022-01273-1
32. Katz, J., Crean, H. F., Cerulli, C., & Poleshuck, E. L. (2018). Material hardship and mental health symptoms among a predominantly low income sample of pregnant women seeking prenatal care. *Maternal and Child Health Journal, 22*(9), 1360–1367. https://doi.org/10.1007/s10995-018-2518-x
33. Qobadi, M., Collier, C., & Zhang, L. (2016). The effect of stressful life events on postpartum depression: Findings from the 2009–2011 Mississippi pregnancy risk assessment monitoring system. *Maternal and Child Health Journal, 20*(1), 164–172. https://doi.org/10.1007/s10995-016-2028-7

34. Reid, K. M., & Taylor, M. G. (2015). Stress and maternal postpartum depression: The importance of stress type and timing. *Population Research and Policy Review*, *34*(6), 851–875. https://doi.org/10.1007/s11113-015-9368-7
35. Richards, M., Weigel, M., Li, M., Rosenberg, M., & Ludema, C. (2020). Household food insecurity and antepartum depression in the National Children's Study. *Annals of Epidemiology*, *44*, 38–44. https://doi.org/10.1016/j.annepidem.2020.01.010
36. Ruyak, S. L., Flores-Montoya, A., & Boursaw, B. (2017). Antepartum services and symptoms of postpartum depression in at-risk women. *Journal of Obstetric, Gynecologic & Neonatal Nursing*, *46*(5), 696–708. https://doi.org/10.1016/j.jogn.2017.07.006
37. Sampson, M., Duron, J. F., Mauldin, R. L., Kao, D., & Davidson, M. (2017). Postpartum depression, risk factors, and child's home environment among mothers in a home visiting program. *Journal of Child and Family Studies*, *26*(10), 2772–2781. https://doi.org/10.1007/s10826-017.0783-8
38. Stone, S. L., Diop, H., Declercq, E., Cabral, H. J., Fox, M. P., & Wise, L. A. (2015). Stressful events during pregnancy and postpartum depressive symptoms. *Journal of Women's Health*, *24*(5), 384–393. https://doi.org/10.1089/jwh.2014.4857
39. Lafferty, A. K., Duryea, E., Martin, R., Moseley, L., Lopez, M., McIntire, D. D., Spong, C. Y., & Nelson, D. B. (2024). A prospective study of social needs associated with mental health among postpartum patients living in underserved communities. *American Journal of Perinatology*, *41*(S 01), e2396–e2402. https://doi.org/10.1055/a-2113-2739
40. Clarke, L. S., Riley, H. E., Corwin, E. J., Dunlop, A. L., & Hogue, C. J. R. (2022). The unique contribution of gendered racial stress to depressive symptoms among pregnant Black women. *Women's Health*, *18*, 17455057221104657. https://doi.org/10.1177/17455057221104657
41. Segre, L. S., Mehner, B. T., & Brock, R. L. (2021). Perceived racial discrimination and depressed mood in perinatal women: An extension of the Domain Specific Stress Index. *Women's Health Issues*, *31*(3), 254–262. https://doi.org/10.1016/j.whi.2020.12.008
42. Chavez, L. J., Tyson, D. P., Davenport, M. A., Kelleher, K. J., & Chisolm, D. J. (2023). Social needs as a risk factor for positive postpartum depression screens in pediatric primary care. *Academic Pediatrics*, *23*(7), 1411–1416. https://doi.org/10.1016/j.acap.2023.03.007
43. Bossick, A. S., Bossick, N. R., Callegari, L. S., Carey, C. M., Johnson, H., & Katon, J. G. (2022). Experiences of racism and postpartum depression symptoms, care-seeking, and diagnosis. *Archives of Women's Mental Health*, *25*(4), 717–727. https://doi.org/10.1007/s00737-022-01232-w
44. Dekel, S., Ein-Dor, T., Berman, Z., Barsoumian, I. S., Agarwal, S., & Pitman, R. K. (2019). Delivery mode is associated with maternal mental health following childbirth. *Archives of Women's Mental Health*, *22*(6), 817–824. https://doi.org/10.1007/s00737-019-00968-2
45. Lewkowitz, A. K., Rosenbloom, J. I., Keller, M., López, J. D., Macones, G. A., Olsen, M. A., & Cahill, A. G. (2019). Association between severe maternal morbidity and psychiatric illness within 1 year of hospital discharge after delivery. *Obstetrics & Gynecology*, *134*(4), 695–707. https://doi.org/10.1097/AOG.0000000000003434
46. Bay, F., & Sayiner, F. D. (2021). Perception of traumatic childbirth of women and its relationship with postpartum depression. *Women & Health*, *61*(5), 479–489. https://doi.org/10.1080/03630242.2021.1927287
47. Jiang, T., Tuxunjiang, X., Wumaier, G., Li, X., & Li, L. (2022). Path analysis of influencing factors for prenatal depressive symptoms in pregnant women. *Journal of Affective Disorders*, *317*, 397–402. https://doi.org/10.1016/j.jad.2022.08.076
48. Waller, R., Kornfield, S. L., White, L. K., Chaiyachati, B. H., Barzilay, R., Njoroge, W., Parish-Morris, J., Duncan, A., Himes, M. M., Rodriguez, Y., Seidlitz, J., Riis, V., Burris, H. H., Gur, R. E., & Elovitz, M. A. (2022). Clinician-reported childbirth outcomes, patient-reported childbirth trauma, and risk for postpartum depression. *Archives of Women's Mental Health*, *25*(5), 985–993. https://doi.org/10.1007/s00737-022-01263-3
49. eClinicalMedicine (2024). Safeguarding maternal mental health in the perinatal period. *eClinicalMedicine*, *71*, 102663. https://doi.org/10.1016/j.eclinm.2024.102663
50. Wohrer, F., Ngo, H., DiDomenico, J., Ma, X., Roberts, M. H., & Bakhireva, L. N. (2024). Potentially modifiable risk and protective factors affecting mental and emotional wellness in pregnancy. *Frontiers in Human Neuroscience*, *18*. https://doi.org/10.3389/fnhum.2024.1323297

51. Hofheimer, J. A., McGowan, E. C., Smith, L. M., Meltzer-Brody, S., Carter, B. S., Dansereau, L. M., Pastyrnak, S., Helderman, J. B., Neal, C. R., DellaGrotta, S. A., O'Shea, T. M. D., & Lester, B. M. (2024). Risk factors for postpartum depression and severe distress among mothers of very preterm infants at NICU discharge. *American Journal of Perinatology, 41*(10), 1396–1408. https://doi.org/10.1055/s-0043-1768132
52. Nelson, T., Ernst, S. C., & Watson-Singleton, N. N. (2023). Perinatal complications, poor hospital treatment, and positive screen for postpartum depressive symptoms among Black women. *Journal of Racial and Ethnic Health Disparities, 10*(3), 1371–1378. https://doi.org/10.1007/s40615-022-01322-6
53. Adaji, R., Wheeler, J. M., Misra, D. P., & Giurgescu, C. (2023). Mother-father relationship and depressive symptoms among pregnant Black women. *Western Journal of Nursing Research, 45*(11), 1027–1034. https://doi.org/10.1177/01939459231202725
54. Feinberg, E., Declercq, E., Lee, A., & Belanoff, C. (2022). The relationship between social support and postnatal anxiety and depression: Results from the listening to mothers in California survey. *Women's Health Issues, 32*(3), 251–260. https://doi.org/10.1016/j.whi.2022.01.005
55. Adlington, K., Vasquez, C., Pearce, E., Wilson, C. A., Nowland, R., Taylor, B. L., Spring, S., & Johnson, S. (2023). "Just snap out of it" – the experience of loneliness in women with perinatal depression: A meta-synthesis of qualitative studies. *BMC Psychiatry, 23*(1), 110. https://doi.org/10.1186/s12888-023-04532-2
56. Ponzini, G. T., Snider, M. D. H., Evey, K. J., & Steinman, S. A. (2021). Women's knowledge of postpartum anxiety disorders, depression, and cognitive behavioral therapy. *The Journal of Nervous and Mental Disease, 209*(6), 426–433. https://doi.org/10.1097/NMD.0000000000001315
57. Leach, L. S., Poyser, C., & Fairweather-Schmidt, K. (2017). Maternal perinatal anxiety: A review of prevalence and correlates. *Clinical Psychologist, 21*(1), 4–19. https://doi.org/10.1111/cp.12058
58. Fairbrother, N., Janssen, P., Antony, M. M., Tucker, E., & Young, A. H. (2016). Perinatal anxiety disorder prevalence and incidence. *Journal of Affective Disorders, 200*, 148–155. https://doi.org/10.1016/j.jad.2015.12.082
59. Fawcett, E. J., Fairbrother, N., Cox, M. L., White, I. R., & Fawcett, J. M. (2019). The prevalence of anxiety disorders during pregnancy and the postpartum period: A multivariate bayesian meta-analysis. *The Journal of Clinical Psychiatry, 80*(4), 18r12527. https://doi.org/10.4088/JCP.18r12527
60. Kelly-Taylor, K., Badon, S. E., Dyer, W. T., Asera, A., Dong, H., Baker, T., Nance, N., Kershaw, K. N., Quesenberry, C. P., Young-Wolff, K. C., Bhalala, M., Erickson-Ridout, K., & Avalos, L. A. (2024). Racial residential segregation and mental health during pregnancy. *JAMA Health Forum, 5*(10), e243669. https://doi.org/10.1001/jamahealthforum.2024.3669
61. Hall, S. V., Zivin, K., Piatt, G. A., Weaver, A., Tilea, A., Zhang, X., & Moyer, C. A. (2023). Racial disparities in diagnosis of postpartum mood and anxiety disorders among symptomatic Medicaid enrollees, 2012–2015. *Psychiatric Services, 75*(2). https://doi.org/10.1176/appi.ps.20230094
62. Ayers, S., Sinesi, A., Coates, R., Cheyne, H., Maxwell, M., Best, C., McNicol, S., Williams, L. R., Uddin, N., Shakespeare, J., Alderdice, F., & MAP Study Team (2024). When is the best time to screen for perinatal anxiety? A longitudinal cohort study. *Journal of Anxiety Disorders, 103*, 102841. https://doi.org/10.1016/j.janxdis.2024.102841
63. Wenzel, E. S., Gibbons, R. D., O'Hara, M. W., Duffecy, J., & Maki, P. M. (2021). Depression and anxiety symptoms across pregnancy and the postpartum in low-income Black and Latina women. *Archives of Women's Mental Health, 24*(6), 979–986. https://doi.org/10.1007/s00737-021-01139-y
64. van der Zee-van den Berg, A. I., Boere-Boonekamp, M. M., Groothuis-Oudshoorn, C. G. M., & Reijneveld, S. A. (2021). Postpartum depression and anxiety: A community-based study on risk factors before, during and after pregnancy. *Journal of Affective Disorders, 286*, 158–165. https://doi.org/10.1016/j.jad.2021.02.062
65. Seymour-Smith, M., Cruwys, T., Haslam, S. A., & Brodribb, W. (2017). Loss of group memberships predicts depression in postpartum mothers. *Social Psychiatry and Psychiatric Epidemiology, 52*(2), 201–210. https://doi.org/10.1007/s00127-016-1315-3

66. Gelaye, B., Kajeepeta, S., & Williams, M. A. (2016). Suicidal ideation in pregnancy: An epidemiologic review. *Archives of Women's Mental Health, 19*(5), 741–751. https://doi.org/10.1007/s00737-016-0646-0
67. Bodnar-Deren, S., Klipstein, K., Fersh, M., Shemesh, E., & Howell, E. A. (2016). Suicidal ideation during the postpartum period. *Journal of Women's Health, 25*(12), 1219–1224. https://doi.org/10.1089/jwh.2015.5346
68. Kim, J. J., La Porte, L. M., Saleh, M. P., Allweiss, S., Adams, M. G., Zhou, Y., & Silver, R. K. (2015). Suicide risk among perinatal women who report thoughts of self-harm on depression screens. *Obstetrics & Gynecology, 125*(4), 885–893. https://doi.org/10.1097/AOG.0000000000000718
69. Gentile, S. (2011). Suicidal mothers. *Journal of Injury & Violence Research, 3*(2), 90–97. https://doi.org/10.5249/jivr.v3i2.98
70. Zhong, Q. Y., Gelaye, B., Miller, M., Fricchione, G. L., Cai, T., Johnson, P. A., Henderson, C., & Williams, M. A. (2016). Suicidal behavior-related hospitalizations among pregnant women in the USA, 2006–2012. *Archives of Women's Mental Health, 19*(3), 463–472. https://doi.org/10.1007/s00737-015-0597-x
71. Salihu, H. M., Dongarwar, D., Oduguwa, E., Atkinson, J. O., & Harris, T. B. (2022). Racial/ethnic disparity in suicidal ideation, suicide attempt and non-suicidal intentional self-harm among pregnant women in the United States. *Journal of Immigrant and Minority Health, 24*(3), 588–596. https://doi.org/10.1007/s10903-021-01260-1
72. Rodriguez-Cabezas, L., & Clark, C. (2018). Psychiatric emergencies in pregnancy and postpartum. *Clinical Obstetrics and Gynecology, 61*(3), 615–627. https://doi.org/10.1097/GRF.0000000000000377
73. Goldman-Mellor, S., & Margerison, C. E. (2019). Maternal drug-related death and suicide are leading causes of post-partum death in California. *American Journal of Obstetrics and Gynecology*. https://doi.org/10.1016/j.ajog.2019.05.045
74. Orsolini, L., Valchera, A., Vecchiotti, R., Tomasetti, C., Iasevoli, F., Fornaro, M., De Berardis, D., Perna, G., Pompili, M., & Bellantuono, C. (2016). Suicide during perinatal period: Epidemiology, risk factors, and clinical correlates. *Frontiers in Psychiatry, 7*, 138. https://doi.org/10.3389/fpsyt.2016.00138
75. Zhang, L., Yang, Y., Li, M., Zhou, X., Zhang, K., Yin, X., & Liu, H. (2022). The prevalence of suicide ideation and predictive factors among pregnant women in the third trimester. *BMC Pregnancy and Childbirth, 22*(1), 266. https://doi.org/10.1186/s12884-022-04590-6
76. Kitsantas, P., Aljoudi, S. M., Adams, A. R., & Booth, E. J. (2021). Prevalence and correlates of suicidal behaviors during pregnancy: Evidence from the national survey on drug use and health. *Archives of Women's Mental Health, 24*(3), 473–481. https://doi.org/10.1007/s00737-020.01089-x
77. Holman, M. S., & Williams, M. N. (2020). Suicide risk and protective factors: A network approach. *Archives of Suicide Research, 26*(1), 137–154. https://doi.org/10.1080/13811118.2020.1774454
78. Kleiman, E. M., & Liu, R. T. (2013). Social support as a protective factor in suicide: Findings from two nationally representative samples. *Journal of Affective Disorders, 150*(2), 540–545. https://doi.org/10.1016/j.jad.2013.01.033
79. Koire, A., Van Horne, B. S., Nong, Y. H., Cain, C. M., Greeley, C. S., & Puryear, L. (2022). Patterns of peripartum depression screening and detection in a large, multi-site, integrated healthcare system. *Archives of Women's Mental Health, 25*(3), 603–610. https://doi.org/10.1007/s00737-022-01223-x
80. Declercq, E., Feinberg, E., & Belanoff, C. (2022). Racial inequities in the course of treating perinatal mental health challenges: Results from listening to mothers in California. *Birth, 49*(1), 132–140. https://doi.org/10.1111/birt.12584
81. Sidebottom, A., Vacquier, M., LaRusso, E., Erickson, D., & Hardeman, R. (2021). Perinatal depression screening practices in a large health system: Identifying current state and assessing opportunities to provide more equitable care. *Archives of Women's Mental Health, 24*(1), 133–144. https://doi.org/10.1007/s00737-020-01035-x
82. ACOG Committee Opinion (2018, November). *Screening for perinatal depression*. www.acog.org/-/media/project/acog/acogorg/clinical/files/committee-opinion/articles/2018/11/screening-for-perinatal-depression.pdf

83. Prevatt, B. S., & Desmarais, S. L. (2018). Facilitators and barriers to disclosure of postpartum mood disorder symptoms to a healthcare provider. *Maternal and Child Health Journal*, *22*(1), 120–129. https://doi.org/10.1007/s10995-017-2361-5
84. Lawson, A., Dalfen, A., Murphy, K. E., Milligan, N., & Lancee, W. (2019). Use of text messaging for postpartum depression screening and information provision. *Psychiatric Services*, *70*(5), 389–395. https://doi.org/10.1176/appi.ps.201800269
85. Walker, L. O., Sterling, B. S., Becker, H., Hendrickson, S., & Xie, B. (2018). Development and evaluation of a mother-centered toolkit for postpartum behavioral and psychosocial health. *Journal of Behavioral Medicine*, *41*(5), 591–599. https://doi.org/10.1007/s10865-018-9928-5
86. Policy Center for Maternal Mental Health (n.d.). *Maternal mental health screening and tools.* https://policycentermmh.org/screening-overview/
87. American College of Obstetricians and Gynecologists (2024). *Implementing perinatal mental health screening.* www.acog.org/programs/perinatal-mental-health/implementing-perinatal-mental-health-screening
88. Byatt, N., Xiao, R. S., Dinh, K. H., & Waring, M. E. (2016). Mental health care use in relation to depressive symptoms among pregnant women in the USA. *Archives of Women's Mental Health*, *19*(1), 187–191. https://doi.org/10.1007/s00737-015-0524-1
89. Glasheen, C., Colpe, L., Hoffman, V., & Warren, L. K. (2015). Prevalence of serious psychological distress and mental health treatment in a national sample of pregnant and postpartum women. *Maternal and Child Health Journal*, *19*(1), 204–216. https://doi.org/10.1007/s10995-014-1511-2
90. Salameh, T. N., Hall, L. A., Crawford, T. N., Staten, R. R., & Hall, M. T. (2020). Likelihood of mental health and substance use treatment receipt among pregnant women in the USA. *International Journal of Mental Health and Addiction*, 1–17. https://doi.org/10.1007/s11469-020-00247-7
91. Sanmartin, M. X., Ali, M. M., Chen, J., & Dwyer, D. S. (2019). Mental health treatment and unmet mental health care need among pregnant women with major depressive episode in the United States. *Psychiatric Services*, *70*(6), 503–506. https://doi.org/10.1176/appi.ps.201800433
92. Chang, J. J., Tabet, M., Elder, K., Kiel, D. W., & Flick, L. H. (2016). Racial/ethnic differences in the correlates of mental health services use among pregnant women with depressive symptoms. *Maternal and Child Health Journal*, *20*(9), 1911–1922. https://doi.org/10.1007/s10995-016-2005-1
93. Avalos, L. A., Nance, N., Iturralde, E., Badon, S. E., Quesenberry, C. P., Sterling, S., Li, D. K., & Flanagan, T. (2023). Racial-ethnic differences in treatment initiation for new diagnoses of perinatal depression. *Psychiatric Services*, *74*(4), 341–348. https://doi.org/10.1176/appi.ps.20220173
94. Canty, H. R., Sauter, A., Zuckerman, K., Cobian, M., & Grigsby, T. (2019). Mothers' perspectives on follow-up for postpartum depression screening in primary care. *Journal of Developmental & Behavioral Pediatrics*, *40*(2), 139–143. https://doi.org/10.1097/DBP.0000000000000628
95. Young, C. A., Burnett, H., Ballinger, A., Castro, G., Steinberg, S., Nau, M., Bakken, E. H., Thomas, M., & Beck, A. L. (2019). Embedded maternal mental health care in a pediatric primary care clinic: A qualitative exploration of mothers' experiences. *Academic Pediatrics*, *19*(8), 934–941. https://doi.org/10.1016/j.acap.2019.08.004
96. Vanderkruik, R., Freeman, M. P., Claypoole, L. D., Arakelian, M., Kaimal, A. J., Nadel, H., & Cohen, L. S. (2021). Postpartum depression screening: Treatment engagement, barriers to care, and change in depressive symptoms. *Annals of Clinical Psychiatry*, *33*(4), 7–14. https://doi.org/10.12788/acp.0044
97. Beck, C. T. (2023). Experiences of postpartum depression in women of color. *The American Journal of Maternal Child Nursing*, *48*(2), 88–95. https://doi.org/10.1097/NMC.0000000000000889
98. Hanson, M. N., Reese, S., & Newcomer, S. R. (2023). Challenges in accessing mental health care during pregnancy and postpartum in rural Montana. *The American Journal of Maternal Child Nursing*, *48*(5), 252–257. https://doi.org/10.1097/NMC.0000000000000937

99. Dagher, R. K., Pérez-Stable, E. J., & James, R. S. (2021). Socioeconomic and racial/ethnic disparities in postpartum consultation for mental health concerns among US mothers. *Archives of Women's Mental Health*, *24*(5), 781–791. https://doi.org/10.1007/s00737-021-01132-5
100. Jones, A. (2022). Postpartum help-seeking: The role of stigma and mental health literacy. *Maternal and Child Health Journal*, *26*(5), 1030–1037. https://doi.org/10.1007/s10995-022-03399-1
101. Albaugh, A. S., Friedman, S. H., Yang, S. N., & Rosenthal, M. (2018). Attendance at mental health appointments by women who were referred during pregnancy or the postpartum period. *Journal of Obstetric, Gynecologic & Neonatal Nursing*, *47*(1), 3–11. https://doi.org/10.1016/j.jogn.2017.11.001
102. Cluxton-Keller, F., Williams, M., Buteau, J., Donnelly, C. L., Stolte, P., Monroe-Cassel, M., & Bruce, M. L. (2018). Video-delivered family therapy for home visited young mothers with perinatal depressive symptoms: Quasi-experimental implementation-effectiveness hybrid trial. *JMIR Mental Health*, *5*(4), e11513. https://doi.org/10.2196/11513
103. Cook, C., Goyal, D., & Allen, M. (2019). Experiences of women with postpartum depression participating in a support group led by mental health providers. *MCN: The American Journal of Maternal/Child Nursing*, *44*(4), 228–233. https://doi.org/10.1097/NMC.0000000000000533
104. Diebold, A., Segovia, M., Johnson, J. K., Degillio, A., Zakieh, D., Park, H. J., Lim, K., & Tandon, S. D. (2020). Acceptability and appropriateness of a perinatal depression preventive group intervention: A qualitative analysis. *BMC Health Services Research*, *20*(1), 1–12. https://doi.org/10.1186/s12913-020-5031-z
105. Smith, M. V., & Kruse-Austin, A. (2015). A gender-informed model to train community health workers in maternal mental health. *Evaluation and Program Planning*, *51*, 59–62. https://doi.org/10.1016/j.evalprogplan.2014.12.008
106. Byatt, N., Biebel, K., Simas, T. A. M., Sarvet, B., Ravech, M., Allison, J., & Straus, J. (2016). Improving perinatal depression care: The Massachusetts child psychiatry access project for moms. *General Hospital Psychiatry*, *40*, 12–17. https://doi.org/10.1016/j.genhosppsych.2016.03.002
107. Pedersen, S. C., Maindal, H. T., & Ryom, K. (2021). "I wanted to be there as a father, but I couldn't": A qualitative study of fathers' experiences of postpartum depression and their help-seeking behavior. *American Journal of Men's Health*, *15*(3), 15579883211024375. https://doi.org/10.1177/15579883211024375
108. Reay, M., Mayers, A., Knowles-Bevis, R., & Knight, M. T. D. (2024). Understanding the barriers fathers face to seeking help for paternal perinatal depression: Comparing fathers to men outside the perinatal period. *International Journal of Environmental Research and Public Health*, *21*(1), 16. https://doi.org/10.3390/ijerph21010016
109. Álvarez-García, P., García-Fernández, R., Martín-Vázquez, C., Calvo-Ayuso, N., & Quiroga-Sánchez, E. (2024). Postpartum depression in fathers: A systematic review. *Journal of Clinical Medicine*, *13*(10), 2949. https://doi.org/10.3390/jcm13102949
110. Goodman, J. H. (2004). Paternal postpartum depression, its relationship to maternal postpartum depression, and implications for family health. *Journal of Advanced Nursing*, *45*(1), 26–35. https://doi.org/10.1046/j.1365-2648.2003.02857.x
111. Wells, M. B., & Jeon, L. (2023). Paternal postpartum depression, coparenting, and father-infant bonding: Testing two mediated models using structural equation modeling. *Journal of Affective Disorders*, *325*, 437–443. https://doi.org/10.1016/j.jad.2022.12.163
112. Wainwright, S., Caskey, R., Rodriguez, A., Holicky, A., Wagner-Schuman, M., & Glassgow, A. E. (2023). Screening fathers for postpartum depression in a maternal-child health clinic: A program evaluation in a midwest urban academic medical center. *BMC Pregnancy and Childbirth*, *23*(1), 675. https://doi.org/10.1186/s12884-023-05966-y
113. Mayo Clinic (2022). *Postpartum depression*. www.mayoclinic.org/diseases-conditions/postpartum-depression/symptoms-causes/syc-20376617

4 Substance Use During Pregnancy and the Postpartum Period

Self-Care Moment

Take a moment to notice how your body is feeling. What thoughts are you having? How can you take care of yourself right now? Consider hydrating, grabbing a nourishing snack, or standing up to stretch before reading this chapter.

In the United States, an estimated 5–16% of pregnancies are affected by substance use, and in some areas more than one-quarter of individuals report substance use during the postpartum period.[1,2] Substance use, especially when it rises to the level of a diagnosable substance use disorder (SUD), is a serious condition that often occurs alongside other mental health or social stressors.[3,4] Substance use during pregnancy and the postpartum period can have significant negative effects on physical and mental health – including death from overdose or other complications.[5,6,7]

This chapter focuses on the ways in which community and social service providers can help to identify and support those who are struggling with substance use during pregnancy or the postpartum period. It includes a discussion of research on this topic, practice implications for your work, and reflections on your role as a community or social service provider. Throughout this chapter, you will also hear the stories of Kim, a mother persevering through substance use, and both the Families In Recovery SupporT (FIRST) Steps Together program and the PAT Peer Recovery Model, which aim to support families affected by substance use during pregnancy and the postpartum period.

Key Terms

Substance misuse: "The use of a substance for a purpose not consistent with legal or medical guidelines," such as drugs, tobacco, or alcohol.[8 (p.2)]

Substance use disorder (SUD): "A chronic and progressive disease characterized by an individual's inability to control their use of drugs or alcohol, despite negative effects and consequences."[8 (p.2)]

Addiction: "The most severe form of . . . SUD. It is a compulsive craving for a substance."[8 (p.3)]

DOI: 10.4324/9781003476474-4

A Note About Language

There is a great deal of stigma and misinformation around substance use in society. Those who struggle with SUDs during pregnancy or the postpartum period are often harshly judged by society. Community and social service providers can help to shift the narrative by using accurate, non-stigmatizing, compassionate, and person-first language when talking about this population. Following are suggestions drawn from the United States National Institute on Drug Abuse.[9]

- Instead of "*addict*" or "*user*," a "*person with substance use disorder*" or "*person with [specific substance] addiction.*"
- Instead of "*substance or drug abuser*," a "*patient*" or "*client.*"
- Instead of "*junkie*," a "*[The person's name] is in active use.*"
- Instead of "*alcoholic*" or "*drunk*" (noun), a "*person who misuses alcohol*" or "*person who engages in unhealthy/hazardous alcohol use*" or "*person with alcohol use disorder.*"
- Instead of "*former/reformed addict*," a "*person in recovery.*"
- Instead of "*substance/drug abuse*" when referring to illicit drugs, "*substance/drug use.*" For prescription medications, "*drug/medication misuse*" or "*drug/medication used other than prescribed.*"
- Instead of "*habit*," a "*substance use disorder*" or "*drug addiction.*"
- Instead of "*clean*" when referring to toxicology screening results, "*testing negative.*" For non-toxicology purposes, "*not currently drinking/using drugs*," "*abstinent from alcohol/drugs*," "*in remission/recovery.*"
- Instead of "*dirty*," a when referring to toxicology screening results, "*testing positive.*" For non-toxicology purposes, "*person who uses drugs.*"
- Instead of "*addicted baby*," a "*baby born to [someone] who used drugs while pregnant*," a "*baby with signs of withdrawal from prenatal drug exposure*," or "*newborn exposed to substances.*"

Stigma and Other Considerations

Substance use affects a significant number of families during pregnancy and the postpartum period; however, it can be difficult to identify those who are affected and to connect them to appropriate supports. Individuals may not disclose that they are struggling with substance use for a variety of reasons, such as fear of judgment, fear of legal consequences (when using illicit substances), fear of involvement with the child welfare system, or lack of awareness of the potential health repercussions of substance use during pregnancy or the postpartum period.[10,11,12,13,14,15,16,17] Therefore, it is important for community and social service providers to: (a) recognize common signs, symptoms, risks, and protective factors for substance use; (b) move away from common myths and biases about substance use and the people who struggle with it; (c) understand the fear and hesitation that their clients may feel about discussing substance use with medical, community, and social service providers; and (d) learn ways to effectively and compassionately raise and discuss this topic.

Relatedly, it is important to understand that while there are numerous factors that increase the risk of substance use (i.e., past substance use history, younger age, life stress and trauma), substance use can affect anyone. For this reason, the American College of Obstetricians and Gynecologists and other entities recommend screening everyone for substance use during pregnancy, not just those with identified risk factors.[18,19] It notes that only screening people with certain risk factors can increase the stigma around substance use and can also result in missing affected individuals.[19]

Many healthcare providers screen pregnant and postpartum patients for substance use; however, community and social service providers are also well-positioned to conduct basic screenings – and in some cases, even better positioned given the strong and trusting relationships that they build over time. Some existing measures such as the 4Ps Plus© screener include screening questions for substance use (i.e., alcohol, tobacco, cannabis, illicit drugs), as well as depression and domestic violence during pregnancy – all of which have been found to co-occur during pregnancy and the postpartum period.[19,20,21,22,23,24,25] Research suggests that it can also be valuable to ask about other household members' substance use – both from a health and safety perspective (i.e., exposure to second-hand smoke, risk of physical contact with other substances or items like needles), and because substance use by other household members (particularly romantic partners) can increase the likelihood that someone will do the same during pregnancy or the postpartum period.[26,27,28,29]

As previously noted, pregnant and postpartum individuals with significant stress, trauma histories, and/or mental health difficulties are more likely to struggle with substance use than those who do not have these risk factors.[30,31,32] It is also common for people to co-use multiple substances (i.e., alcohol, tobacco, other drugs).[33] Those who struggle with substance use are also less likely to receive standard prenatal care and frequently report challenges in accessing specialized treatments for substance use and/or mental health disorders.[10,34,35,36,37] Lower rates of healthcare access have been linked to many factors including lack of transportation, financial and insurance coverage issues, previous negative experiences with healthcare providers, and fear.[38] This underscores the importance of providing quality referrals and, perhaps most importantly, social and emotional support to help people access the healthcare and support services that they need.

In the following sections of this chapter, we will focus on four of the substances more commonly used during pregnancy and the postpartum period: opioids, cannabis, alcohol, and tobacco/nicotine. Regrettably, space limitations preclude us from discussing other types of substance use in depth. Readers should also keep in mind that some individuals may use multiple substances during pregnancy or the postpartum period, particularly if they were engaging in substance use in the year before getting pregnant and/or if they are younger than 25.[33,39,40,41]

Putting It Into Practice

- ***Sensitively screen for substance use during pregnancy, as well as the postpartum period.*** Experts agree that screening for depression, anxiety, and substance use should be universal during pregnancy, meaning that everyone should receive these screenings. As mentioned, selective screenings (i.e., only screening people that are suspected to be using substances) can contribute to the stigma around substance use and can also lead to missing individuals who are quietly struggling with these issues. Continuing screenings during the postpartum period is also wise, given that that this is often a period of increased stress and risk of relapse.

Even if a client has been screened by their healthcare provider, it can still be valuable for community and social service providers to conduct their own screenings. Community and social service providers typically see clients more often than healthcare providers, and because of the trusting relationships that are characteristic of these service delivery methods, clients may be more comfortable opening up honestly about their substance use with them.
Stigma around SUD can cause pregnant and postpartum clients to feel reluctant about disclosing their struggles. Increase their comfort by conveying a warm, supportive, and non-judgmental attitude.

- ***Provide education about the importance of abstaining from substances during pregnancy and breast feeding.*** Provide clear, supportive guidance to all pregnant and postpartum clients about the importance of talking to their healthcare provider about the safety of any prescription or non-prescription drugs they may be taking, as well as abstaining from substances like alcohol, tobacco, and nicotine products. One way to start these conversations is by asking clients what they have heard about this topic from various sources (i.e., their healthcare provider, friends, family, social media), and about any relevant cultural beliefs or practices. From there, the provider can sensitively ask follow-up questions about the client's past and current history with substances, address any misconceptions, and connect the client with appropriate resources if needed.
- ***Address the interconnectedness of substance use with other issues.*** SUD is often interconnected with or influenced by other issues. Therefore, it can be very helpful to develop a holistic picture of your clients' experiences, with an eye on identifying those who may be at increased risk for substance use during or after pregnancy. This includes identifying recent and current mental health symptoms (i.e., using a standardized screening tool to assess for current depression and anxiety symptoms), but also asking about past mental health and trauma history. You are most likely to obtain accurate information about these sensitive topics when you have already cultivated trusting, responsive working relationships with your clients.

Another important factor to assess is substance use by other individuals in your pregnant or postpartum client's life and home – particularly romantic partners. Continued exposure to substances can make abstaining more challenging during and after pregnancy. Furthermore, pregnant and postpartum individuals whose partners are struggling with substance use may be at increased risk for experiencing domestic violence, financial difficulties, or other struggles. When possible, it is valuable to take a "whole-family" approach to this work – collaborating with both parents and other caregivers to create a safe, supportive, substance-free pregnancy and environment for their baby.

Take Time to Reflect

What sorts of messages have you heard about people who struggle with substance use? For example, what kinds of things did you hear at home, at school, or in your community when you were growing up? What about in the media or at work? Consider whether any of these messages might be out of date or harmful to people struggling with substance use. If so, what can you do to promote less judgmental, more compassionate ways of thinking, talking, and working with this group?

Kim's Story ∞

Kim, a 32-year-old woman from Michigan, recently shared her story of persevering through substance use in a *New York Times* article.[42] Kim survived a chaotic, abusive childhood, and began to struggle with substance use and housing instability as a teenager. As a young adult, she made 17 attempts at recovery but relapsed in the absence of adequate medical and social support. When she became pregnant with her first child, she was struggling with addiction to methamphetamines, alcohol, and anti-anxiety medication. Motivated to make a change for herself and her baby, she enrolled in a program that provides coordinated obstetric care and substance use treatment. To her huge credit, she gave birth to a healthy baby boy. Unfortunately, amidst the stresses of the transition to parenthood, Kim relapsed and her son was placed in foster care at 6 months old. In her despair, she fell deeper into substance use. Yet, when she became pregnant with her second child a few months later, she was once again motivated to try to make a positive change. She returned to treatment, moved into a sober house, started therapy, got a job, and participated in supervised visits with her son. The article containing Kim's story ends with a picture of her with a pregnant belly, gazing lovingly at her son and helping him take baby steps.

Opioid Use During Pregnancy and Postpartum

There is a growing epidemic of opioid misuse in the United States and beyond.[43] In some cases, people are initially prescribed a strong opioid drug (i.e., morphine, oxycodone, hydrocodone, fentanyl) by a healthcare provider for pain management, and then go on to use it in ways other than how it was prescribed (i.e., in larger doses, for longer periods of time, or for different reasons than prescribed). In other cases, individuals may obtain opioid drugs such as the ones just listed, among others (i.e., heroin), in non-medical settings and become addicted.[19,44] Opioid use can quickly devolve into opioid use disorder, which includes symptoms such as physical dependence (i.e., withdrawal symptoms when stopping the drug, needing heavier or more frequent doses to get the same high), strong physical and emotional cravings, increasingly dangerous risk-taking to obtain the drug, physical health symptoms (i.e., weight loss, drowsiness), and relationship problems. People with opioid use disorder often need medical supervision and treatment to withdraw safely. In the most tragic cases, people can die from overdosing, from consuming contaminated drugs, or from health complications related to chronic opioid misuse.

Opioid use during pregnancy can be very risky for these reasons, and because it has been linked to higher rates of preeclampsia, preterm delivery, health complications, and maternal and infant death.[45] According to the CDC, about 7% of pregnant individuals are prescribed opioid drugs by their healthcare providers for pain management or other health conditions, and about 20% of this group reports misusing these drugs during pregnancy.[46] The latter group includes individuals who were already struggling with risky opioid use before pregnancy, as well as individuals who began engaging in risky opioid use during pregnancy. Meanwhile, according to researchers at the U.S. National Institutes of Health, the number of drug overdose-related deaths during pregnancy and the postpartum period has significantly increased in recent years, with the highest increases occurring among those between the ages of 35 and 44.[47] In this group, the average overdose death rate was 16 out of 100,000 in 2021.[47] For individuals who have been prescribed opioid drugs for pain management during the postpartum months, obtaining multiple prescription refills has been linked to increased risk of death.[48]

Anyone can struggle with opioid use, regardless of age, gender, race, ethnicity, socio-economic status, educational background, or other factors. With that being said, research studies have found that opioid misuse tends to be higher in rural areas, among people with lower levels of educational attainment, and among people struggling with food and housing insecurity, depression, and intimate partner violence.[24,45,49,50,51,52] The "cause and effect" relationship between these experiences can go in both directions – for example, people who are struggling financially and mentally may turn to opioids as a coping strategy; or alternatively, people using opioids may struggle to manage their day-to-day life, jobs, and relationships, increasing their risk of financial and mental health problems.

The good news is that there are effective treatments for opioid misuse, though they can sometimes be difficult to access – particularly in rural areas. Typically, the frontline is medication-assisted treatment (MAT), in which a medical professional provides medication that helps the person cope with opioid withdrawal symptoms and avoid relapse.[19] The American College of Obstetricians and Gynecologists cites the following several reasons why MAT is often a preferred treatment for those struggling with substance use disorder in pregnancy.[19]

- "[MAT] prevents opioid withdrawal symptoms and has been shown to prevent complications of nonmedical opioid use by reducing relapse risk and its associated consequences";
- "It also improves adherence to prenatal care and addiction treatment programs"; and
- "[MAT] in combination with prenatal care has been demonstrated to reduce the risk of obstetric complications."

It is often recommended that people who participated in MAT while pregnant continue treatment after giving birth, because the stress of the postpartum period can increase the risk of opioid use relapse.[19,53]

Many infants who were exposed to substances in utero exhibit neonatal abstinence syndrome (NAS) after birth. This is also true for infants born to individuals who participated in MAT while pregnant, with substantial numbers of these infants exhibiting NAS. Infants with NAS may exhibit a range of symptoms – for example, irritability, difficulty sleeping, high-pitched crying, and poor sucking reflexes resulting in difficulty feeding.[19] These symptoms usually appear within three days of birth (though they can take as long as two weeks to emerge), and typically last anywhere between a few days and a few weeks. Infants with NAS may require additional interventions or treatment, and their families often benefit from extra education and support as well (see "Putting It Into Practice" following). Therefore, it is important that healthcare providers whose pregnant patients are struggling with substance use (i.e., their obstetric and SUD treatment teams) collaborate with the baby's healthcare team before birth to prepare for the possibility of NAS.

In addition to MAT, psychotherapy and community support services can be helpful additions to a comprehensive plan of care for those struggling with substance use during pregnancy and the postpartum period, particularly for those who are also experiencing mental health or financial difficulties.[54,55]

Putting It Into Practice

- ***Reduce stigma around SUD treatment.*** Some people may believe that there is a stigma around certain treatment approaches in pregnancy, particularly MAT for opioid use disorder. Support pregnant and postpartum clients and their families in feeling more confident about MAT by repeating and reinforcing information provided by the healthcare provider and other reputable sources. For example, talk with families about evidence that attempting abstinence (i.e., going "cold turkey") is often unsuccessful, and that relapsing can have health consequences for both them and their baby. Share that MAT, when combined with prenatal care, has been shown to reduce the risk of obstetric complications.[19]

  As with other aspects of prenatal care, you may also need to help connect your pregnant or postpartum client to culturally responsive and supportive treatment facilities. Unfortunately, treatment options are often far away or otherwise difficult to obtain, particularly in rural areas. In these situations, work with the client and their family to problem-solve around these barriers (i.e., identifying transportation or childcare options). Meanwhile, if a pregnant or postpartum client encounters difficulties or insensitivities once they are in treatment, support them around self-advocacy and, as needed or requested, offer additional advocacy on their behalf.

- ***Provide education and support around NAS.*** Individuals who have struggled with using opioids or similar substances during pregnancy are at increased risk of giving birth to babies with NAS. These parents often experience complex emotions such as guilt, fear, or sadness. In these situations, community and social service providers can make a difference by helping to prepare clients and their families for what they might expect upon their baby's birth – for example, symptoms the infant may display, typical treatment approaches, and strategies the family can use to soothe the baby (i.e., lessening light and sound stimulation, swaddling, gentle rocking, rooming in with the parent). They can also help parents develop a list of questions for their healthcare provider and their baby's healthcare provider.

  Breastfeeding has been found to be helpful for infants with NAS, provided that the individual breastfeeding is receiving stable treatment, not using illicit drugs, and does not have any other medical contraindications for breastfeeding. Support clients in considering whether they would like to breastfeed, and if so, provide supportive education and resources, including a referral to a skilled lactation consultant.

It is also important to be familiar with the protocols of local healthcare and legal systems for reporting instances of newborns believed to have been exposed to drugs or alcohol. For example, in the United States, guided by the Child Abuse Prevention and Treatment Act (CAPTA),

> most states direct healthcare providers to report infants who present with symptoms consistent with prenatal exposure to drugs or alcohol to child protective services . . . . Many states specify that a report of NAS to [child protective services] is not a de facto finding of child abuse or neglect, an approach taken to dissociate involvement of [child protective services] from punitive measures and to incentivize providers to make the referral.[56]

You should also be informed about how your state handles Plans of Safe Care, or "Family Care Plans," a related requirement of CAPTA. These plans are "designed to ensure the safety and well-being of an infant with prenatal substance exposure by addressing the health and SUD treatment needs of both the infant and the affected family or caregiver."[57] In many locales, the services provided by community and social service providers are integrated into the plan.

Take Action

Even if you are not a medical provider, it is important to know the signs and symptoms of a possible opioid overdose. According to the National Harm Reduction Coalition,[58] these can include the following.

- Being awake but unable to talk
- Loss of consciousness
- Unresponsiveness to being touched
- Changes in skin tone (bluish purple for lighter-skinned people; gray or ashen for darker-skinned people)
- Changes in fingernail and lip color (blue or purplish black)
- Choking or gurgling sounds
- Vomiting
- Limp body
- Pale or clammy face
- Breathing very slowly, shallowly, or erratically, or not breathing at all
- Slow or erratic pulse/heartbeat; or no pulse at all

If you are at all suspicious that someone is overdosing, provide emergency first aid and/or naloxone if you carry it, and contact emergency medical services. Overdoses can be fatal, so it is always better to be safe than sorry.

Take Action

Did you know that in many regions, anyone can carry and administer naloxone? Naloxone is a fast-acting, life-saving medicine that can temporarily restore normal breathing to a person who is experiencing an opioid overdose. It can be administered by anyone, not just medical professionals, as a nasal spray or as an injection. Consider talking to your local pharmacist or healthcare provider about getting a dose of naloxone to keep with you at all times. Some communities and local organizations also have special naloxone programs through which you can access materials and trainings for low to no cost.

Cannabis Use During Pregnancy and Postpartum

Use of cannabis (i.e., marijuana, weed) is increasingly common in the general population, especially since many regions are now legalizing its use for both medical and recreational purposes. However, leading healthcare organizations advise that it is important to stop using cannabis when trying to conceive, or, in the case of unexpected pregnancy, as soon as the pregnancy is discovered.[59,60] This is because cannabis use can negatively affect fertility, and because cannabis use during pregnancy has been linked to many health risks for the developing baby, such as preterm birth, fetal growth restriction, abnormal brain development, stillbirth, and longer-term difficulties with executive functioning and behavior.[61,62,63] Cannabis use is also discouraged during the postpartum period because of the risks of impaired caregiving, transmission through breastmilk, and second-hand smoke exposure for infants.

Nevertheless, many individuals find it difficult to stop using cannabis during pregnancy for physical, emotional, or social reasons. Others start using cannabis during pregnancy as a way of coping with stress or pregnancy-related physical discomfort, including nausea.[28,64] Those who use cannabis frequently or at high doses may experience unpleasant withdrawal symptoms when they try to quit, such as anxiety, sleep difficulties, gastrointestinal symptoms, and intense cravings. Furthermore, research shows that many people do not realize the risks associated with cannabis use during pregnancy.[12,13,65,66] For example, one study found that, in a group of both pregnant and non-pregnant women, about 70% thought there was little or no risk to using cannabis once or twice a week.[13] In this group, 4% of pregnant women reported using cannabis in the past month, and 18% of these women met diagnostic criteria for cannabis dependence or disorder.[13] These findings generally align with other estimates of cannabis use during pregnancy.[67,68]

Research has found that, in the United States, several groups are more likely to use cannabis during pregnancy, including those who are non-Hispanic White, who are unmarried, who have less than the equivalent of a 12th grade education, and/or who also use tobacco, alcohol, or illicit drugs.[13,68] However, given changing beliefs and practices related to cannabis use in society at large, it would likely be helpful to provide information and screenings to all clients during pregnancy and the postpartum period. In holding these discussions, community and social service providers should take a compassionate, sensitive, and non-judgmental stance, keeping in mind the complicated history of how cannabis use has been perceived and addressed in recent decades.[69]

Alcohol Use During Pregnancy and Postpartum

Alcohol is a legal and commonly used substance around the world; however, leading healthcare organizations advise that it is important to stop consuming alcohol when one is trying to conceive, or, in the case of unexpected pregnancy, as soon as the pregnancy is discovered. Alcohol use during pregnancy has been linked to a variety of adverse birth outcomes, such as preterm birth, birth defects, low birthweight, neurodevelopmental disabilities (i.e., fetal alcohol spectrum disorders [FASD]), and stillbirth, as well as increased risk of sudden unexpected infant death syndrome.[70,71] Despite popular misconceptions, the American College of Obstetricians and Gynecologists and others advise that no amount or type of alcohol is safe to consume during pregnancy.[72,73] Even small to moderate levels of alcohol consumption can have negative effects on the developing fetus, and heavy or binge drinking is especially risky.[72,74]

Despite this guidance, many individuals find it difficult to stop drinking alcohol during pregnancy – even if they were only drinking at low or moderate levels before they became pregnant. For those struggling with alcohol use disorder, abstaining from alcohol can be hugely challenging for physical, emotional, and social reasons. For example, people with alcohol use disorder often experiences withdrawal symptoms when they try to stop drinking, particularly if they try to do so quickly in a short period of time (i.e., upon learning about an unexpected pregnancy). Alcohol withdrawal symptoms can range in severity from minor (i.e., headaches, anxiety, difficulty sleeping) to severe (i.e., seizures, hallucinations, alcohol withdrawal delirium [delirium tremens]) to fatal – and in more serious cases, medical supervision and treatment is needed to safely go through withdrawal.[75]

In the United States, recent estimates of the percentage of individuals who drink alcohol during pregnancy have ranged from 8–14%, with about 5% of pregnant individuals reporting recent binge drinking (typically defined as having four or more standard-size drinks in a two-hour period for women).[70] Research has identified several risk factors for alcohol use during pregnancy such as previous drinking history, current tobacco and cannabis use, experiencing intimate partner violence, and depression.[21,22,34] Notably, some individuals who are experiencing depression may turn to alcohol as a coping strategy.[76] One study found that among women struggling with alcohol use, those who also had depression were less likely to change their drinking behavior and more likely to have urges to drink than those who were not depressed.[22]

According to leading healthcare organizations, it is ideal to completely avoid alcohol during pregnancy. However, if this is not possible, the next best scenario is to reduce and stop alcohol consumption as early as possible in pregnancy.[77] With that being said, those who struggle with alcohol use early in pregnancy can still reduce health risks for themselves and their babies by abstaining later in pregnancy. This is where healthcare, community, and social service providers can make a difference by screening all pregnant clients for alcohol use and co-occurring challenges such as intimate partner violence and depression; and by providing information, support, and referrals in compassionate, non-judgmental ways.[78]

During the year after giving birth, many individuals resume drinking alcohol at low or moderate levels.[79] This postpartum period can be a high-risk time for those who had alcohol use disorder before or during pregnancy to relapse, and for those with no previous history to begin drinking heavily as a way of coping with the stress of new parenthood. Heavy drinking during the postpartum period is discouraged because of the risks of impaired caregiving, and because large quantities alcohol can be passed on to breastfeeding babies, with potential short- and long-term effects.[80] Thus, the postpartum period is another important touchpoint for healthcare, community, and social service providers to offer screenings, information, support, and referrals related to alcohol use.

Tobacco and Nicotine Use During Pregnancy and Postpartum

Consuming tobacco and nicotine products (i.e., cigarettes, e-cigarettes, vapes, hookahs) during pregnancy is a significant risk factor for poor health outcomes. Many studies have linked tobacco and nicotine use during pregnancy to increased risk of a wide variety of adverse outcomes such as preeclampsia, placenta abnormalities, restricted fetal growth, birth defects, preterm delivery, stillbirth, and SIDS.[81,82,83,84,85] Meanwhile, tobacco and nicotine use after giving birth has also been linked to adverse maternal and infant outcomes – particularly if the baby is breastfeeding or exposed to second-hand smoke.

According to the CDC, slightly more than half of those who smoked tobacco and nicotine products before pregnancy stopped doing so once they became pregnant. Overall, approximately 5% of pregnant individuals and 7% of postpartum individuals smoke cigarettes.[82] The same research found that certain groups were more likely to smoke tobacco and nicotine products during pregnancy, including those with histories of depression before pregnancy, those with less than the equivalent of a 12th grade education, those living in socioeconomically disadvantaged areas, those with public insurance, and American Indian or Alaska Native individuals (some of whom come from cultures that consider tobacco sacred).[82,86] Meanwhile, use of alternative tobacco and nicotine products (i.e., e-cigarettes, vapes) has become more popular in the general population in recent years and emerging evidence suggests that these products are used at similar or even higher rates than cigarettes during pregnancy and postpartum.[87,88]

Like any substance, tobacco and nicotine can quickly become addictive and very difficult to quit using – underscoring the importance of increasing knowledge and awareness about the risks among all individuals of childbearing age, especially those who are currently pregnant or postpartum. Notably, research suggests that many pregnant and postpartum individuals are not fully aware of the risks of consuming tobacco and nicotine products for themselves and their developing baby. For example, one large survey study found that less than one-quarter of women of childbearing age had strong knowledge of the health risks of smoking during pregnancy.[15] Another survey study found that smokers were less aware of the potential effects of maternal smoking on cancer risk and children's lung development and breathing than non-smokers.[14]

As with alcohol, any reduction in tobacco and nicotine use can reduce the risk of negative health outcomes. While the greatest reductions in risk occur when someone quits using tobacco or nicotine during pregnancy, quitting later in pregnancy or during the postpartum period is also beneficial.[89] Even if it is not possible for someone to quit using tobacco or nicotine products entirely, cutting back on the number of products consumed has been shown to reduce health risks – a finding that many adults do not realize, suggesting that this is important information to advertise.[15] For example, decreasing the total number of cigarettes smoked or the number of times one vapes daily can have a positive impact on both maternal and child health outcomes.

Although quitting tobacco and nicotine use is difficult, there is a great deal of evidence that interventions such as contingency management (a psychosocial intervention that provides rewards and reinforcements for people's efforts to reduce substance use) can be effective.[90] Individuals who have a history of tobacco and nicotine use (before or during pregnancy) also benefit from social and emotional support during and after pregnancy. During the postpartum period, the demands and stressors of welcoming a new baby are major risk factors for relapsing into tobacco and nicotine use – particularly if the postpartum individual is not breastfeeding and thus not concerned about passing on the substance through their breast milk.[91,92] In one study of postpartum former smokers, participants reported that the following strategies helped the most in preventing them from relapsing: "being informed on smoking risks, maintaining goal-oriented thoughts, focusing on their concerns about the baby's health and receiving positive social support from families and friends."[92 (p.140)]

Putting It Into Practice

- ***Emphasize the value of even gradual reductions in substance use, and that it is never too late to quit.*** Advise pregnant clients to abstain from non-prescribed substances, and refer those struggling with significant substance use for professional treatment. In the meantime, convey the important message that even gradual reductions in substance use can have a positive impact on the health of both your client and their developing baby. For example, if the idea of quitting smoking feels too daunting for someone to attempt, they may find it more doable to gradually reduce the number of cigarettes that they smoke each day. In these scenarios, you can become valuable parts of your client's accountability and support team – helping them to stay on track and celebrating their successes. Remember to emphasize to families that, while it is optimal to quit using substances as early in pregnancy as possible, quitting at any point in pregnancy can have a positive impact on overall healthy outcomes. In other words, it is never too late to quit or to seek treatment.

Take Action

In recent years, many new alternative cigarette products (i.e., vapes, e-cigarettes) have entered the market. In fact, many of these products are now more popular than traditional cigarettes, particularly among young people. If you do not know much about these products, take five minutes to conduct an online search to learn more. It can be especially helpful to look up: (a) common terminology or slang related to these products; (b) how these products are used; and (c) the health risks of using these products. Example of search terms you could use are: "vaping information," "what are e-cigarettes," or "vaping terminology."

Families In Recovery SupporT (FIRST) Steps Together and the PAT Peer Recovery Model Δ

Families In Recovery SupporT (FIRST) Steps Together is a free, voluntary peer recovery and parenting support program for pregnant and parenting individuals who are currently struggling with substance use, or who have past histories of challenges in this domain. FIRST Steps Together launched in 2019 in Massachusetts, which has one of the highest prevalence rates of SUD in the United States. Services can be provided in the home, in the community, or online.

FIRST Steps Together pairs current and expecting parents with family recovery support specialists – individuals who have lived experience with substance use and recovery, as well as specialized training. This shared experience creates an authentic, empathetic connection that fosters trust and supports parents' recovery and parenting efforts. As one parent explained while reflecting on what it is like to connect with someone who has had similar struggles:

> If I have somebody reading out of a book . . . I'm not going to want to listen to them. But if somebody is like, 'Hey. I've been there. I've been at my lows, I've been at my highs,' . . . they're more relatable.

FIRST Steps Together also offers a variety of other services aimed at building "recovery and parenting capital," which encompasses the knowledge, skills, and support networks necessary for successful parenting and sustained recovery. Parents can choose to participate in parenting support groups (even after they complete the program, ensuring continued support), care coordination services, and mental health counseling. The program's mental health counselors have specialized training in Mothering from the Inside Out, an intervention designed to strengthen reflective capacity – the ability of parents with SUD to reflect on their own thoughts and emotions and those of their children.

Almost all parents in the program have child welfare involvement, and more than half do not have custody of at least one child at the time of program entry. Parent–child relationships, including during noncustodial family time and reunification, are strengthened through "walking alongside" parents, advocacy, and assistance with planning and concrete needs, all while helping parents stay attuned to their children and themselves.

By addressing community stigma and fostering supportive, non-judgmental relationships, FIRST Steps Together is helping parents build the resilience and confidence they need to succeed in both their recovery and their parenting journey. Workforce development materials on best practices and lessons learned are available online at: https://firststepstogetherma.org/

In addition to FIRST Steps Together, Massachusetts also implements the PAT home visiting model through a peer recovery lens. In the PAT Recovery Coaching model, home visitors with lived experience in substance use and recovery are cross-trained as both PAT home visitors and recovery coaches, and designated as PAT peer recovery specialists. This approach emphasizes relationship-building, participant-driven services, and strengths-based support, which are crucial for overcoming the stigma often associated with SUD.[93]

Your Role as a Community or Social Service Provider

Listening and Learning

The data and information in this chapter present a picture of the substance use challenges that can occur during pregnancy and the postpartum period. Understanding the data, statistics, and stories specific to your community will help you to tailor your services to the issues, needs and strengths of your local community and the families within it. Consider: what do you already know about substance use in your local community (for example, how common it is during pregnancy and the postpartum period, which types of substances are most commonly used)? How can you learn more (i.e., researching information and local data, listening to personal stories of different kinds of families in your community, etc.)?

Advocating

As discussed earlier in this book, your role as a community or service provider operates on two levels: (a) your individual work with families; and (b) your work with systems, including local substance use treatment providers. The lessons outlined in this chapter pertain to both levels of work and point to the need for broader advocacy around supporting pregnant and postpartum clients who are struggling with substance use. You can advocate within your organization – for example, for the development of sensitive, universal substance use screening protocols, for increasing professional development for staff about how to talk with clients about substance use, or for embedding additional support strategies or interventions into your workflow (perhaps including carrying naloxone). You can also advocate outside of your organization in the community at large by lifting up compassionate policies, programs, and initiatives for families affected by substance use.

Take Time to Reflect

Reflecting on the practice implications throughout this chapter and your role as a community or social service provider, what is one area where you believe you are already doing an excellent job? What is one area where you could improve your professional practice or deepen your knowledge and understanding?

Take Action

Now that you have reflected on an area where you could improve your professional practice, create a SMART goal to make it happen. Remember, a SMART goal is, described as follows.

- **S**pecific
- **M**easurable
- **A**chievable
- **R**elevant
- Time-Bound

For example, imagine that you would like to increase your awareness of local facilities that offer MAT during pregnancy and the postpartum period. A SMART goal might be:

> Some of my pregnant and postpartum clients struggle with SUD, and it would be beneficial if I could tell them about local MAT options (**Relevant**). This week

(**Time-Bound**), I will call my state's Health and Human Services Department and conduct online searches for treatment facilities within driving distance (**Specific, Achievable**). I hope to add at least three treatment facilities to our internal referral list by the end of the week. (**Measurable**).

Key Takeaways From This Chapter

1. A significant number of individuals struggle with substance use during and after pregnancy. Substance use affects people from all walks of life, though some groups are at increased risk (i.e., those with past substance use histories or high levels of stressors.) Universal screening, early identification, and effective treatment are essential to promoting healthy outcomes for affected individuals and their babies.
2. It is advisable to abstain from non-prescribed substances during pregnancy and while breastfeeding; however, even gradual reductions in substance use can have positive effects on maternal and infant health. It is never too late to quit and seek support.
3. Community and social service providers can take many steps to support pregnant and postpartum clients who are struggling with substance use, even if they are not healthcare providers. The strong relationships that they build with families over time put them in a strong position to make a difference.

References

1. Forray, A. (2016). Substance use during pregnancy. *F1000Research*, *5*, F1000 Faculty Rev-887. https://doi.org/10.12688/f1000research.7645.1
2. Danielson, M. L., Bohm, M. K., Newsome, K., Claussen, A. H., Kaminski, J. W., Grosse, S. D., Siwakoti, L., Arifkhanova, A., Bitsko, R. H., & Robinson, L. R. (2023). Trends in stimulant prescription fills among commercially insured children and adults – United States, 2016–2021. *Morbidity and Mortality Weekly Report*, *72*, 327–332. https://doi.org/10.15585/mmwr.mm7213a1. Accessed December 2024.
3. Pfeifer, L. R., & Haile, Z. T. (2021). Unmet mental health care needs and illicit drug use during pregnancy. *Journal of Addiction Medicine*, *15*(3), 233–240. https://doi.org/10.1097/ADM.0000000000000752
4. Sujan, A. C., Alexeeff, S. E., Slama, N., Avalos, L. A., Adams, S. R., Conway, A., Ansley, D., & Young-Wolff, K. C. (2023). Patterns of substance use during early pregnancy and associations with behavioral health characteristics. *Journal of Addiction Medicine*, *17*(3), e141–e147. https://doi.org/10.1097/ADM.0000000000001090
5. Courchesne-Krak, N. S., Zúñiga, M. L., Chambers, C., Reed, M. B., Smith, L. R., Ballas, J., & Marienfeld, C. (2023). Substance-related diagnosis type predicts the likelihood and co-occurrence of preterm and cesarean delivery. *Journal of Addictive Diseases*, *41*(2), 137–148. https://doi.org/10.1080/10550887.2022.2082834
6. Nguyen, V. H., & Harley, K. G. (2022). Prenatal cannabis use and infant birth outcomes in the Pregnancy Risk Assessment Monitoring System. *The Journal of Pediatrics*, *240*, 87–93. https://doi.org/10.1016/j.jpeds.2021.08.088
7. Daggy, J. K., Silver, R. M., Guise, D., & Haas, D. M. (2024). The impact of self-reported alcohol, tobacco, and recreational drug use during pregnancy on adverse pregnancy outcomes in first-time mothers. *American Journal of Perinatology*, *41*(10), 1311–1320. https://doi.org/10.1055/s-0042-1753502
8. Maternal, Infant, and Early Childhood Home Visiting (MIECHV). *Understanding the substance use landscape*. Accessed December 2024.

9. National Institute on Drug Abuse (2024). *Words matter – Terms to use and avoid when talking about addiction.* https://nida.nih.gov/nidamed-medical-health-professionals/health-professions-education/words-matter-terms-to-use-avoid-when-talking-about-addiction. Accessed December 2024.
10. Berra, A., Kamo, S., Mohnot, S., Rosselot, J., Suire, A., Stafford, J., Hagan, J., & Stafford, I. (2019). The association between antenatal maternal self-reported substance use, maternal characteristics, and obstetrical variables. *Journal of Addiction Medicine, 13*(6), 464–469. https://doi.org/10.1097/ADM.0000000000000521
11. Jarlenski, M., Tarr, J. A., Holland, C. L., Farrell, D., & Chang, J. C. (2016). Pregnant women's access to information about perinatal marijuana use: A qualitative study. *Women's Health Issues, 26*(4), 452–459. https://doi.org/10.1016/j.whi.2016.03.010
12. Ko, J. Y., Farr, S. L., Tong, V. T., Creanga, A. A., & Callaghan, W. M. (2015). Prevalence and patterns of marijuana use among pregnant and nonpregnant women of reproductive age. *American Journal of Obstetrics and Gynecology, 213*(2), 201-e1. https://doi.org/10.1016/j.ajog.2015.03.021
13. Odibo, I. N., Zamudio, S., Young, J. M., Magann, E. F., & Williams, S. F. (2015). Patient awareness of untoward effects of smoking on fetal and maternal well-being during pregnancy: A pilot study. *Journal of Addiction Medicine, 9*(3), 211–216. https://doi.org/10.1097/ADM.0000000000000119
14. Polen, K. N., Sandhu, P. K., Honein, M. A., Green, K. K., Berkowitz, J. M., Pace, J., & Rasmussen, S. A. (2015). Knowledge and attitudes of adults towards smoking in pregnancy: Results from the HealthStyles© 2008 survey. *Maternal and Child Health Journal, 19*(1), 144–154. https://doi.org/10.1007/s10995-014-1505-0
15. Herriott, A. L. (2024). "I just want the best for him." Pregnancy in the context of substance use disorders: Perspectives of postpartum women. *Birth, 51*(1), 81–88. https://doi.org/10.1111/birt.12761
16. Woodruff, K., Scott, K. A., & Roberts, S. C. M. (2021). Pregnant people's experiences discussing their cannabis use with prenatal care providers in a state with legalized cannabis. *Drug and Alcohol Dependence, 227*, 108998. https://doi.org/10.1016/j.drugalcdep.2021.108998
17. Hilliard, F., Goldstein, E., Nervik, K., Croes, K., Ossorio, P. N., & Zgierska, A. E. (2023). Voices of women with lived experience of substance use during pregnancy: A qualitative study of motivators and barriers to recruitment and retention in research. *Family & Community Health, 46*(1), 1–12. https://doi.org/10.1097/FCH.0000000000000349
18. New York State Office of Addiction Service and Supports (n.d.). *SBIRT: Screening, brief intervention, & referral to treatment.* https://oasas.ny.gov/sbirt
19. The American College of Obstetrician and Gynecologists (2017, August). *Opioid use and opioid use disorder in pregnancy.* www.acog.org/clinical/clinical-guidance/committee-opinion/articles/2017/08/opioid-use-and-opioid-use-disorder-in-pregnancy
20. Deutsch, A. R. (2019). The importance of intimate partner violence in within-relationship and between-person risk for alcohol-exposed pregnancy. *Alcoholism: Clinical and Experimental Research, 43*(4), 679–689. https://doi.org/10.1111/acer.13968
21. Johnson, S. K., von Sternberg, K., & Velasquez, M. M. (2017). A comparison of profiles of transtheoretical model constructs of change among depressed and nondepressed women at risk for an alcohol-exposed pregnancy. *Women's Health Issues, 27*(1), 100–107. https://doi.org/10.1016/j.whi.2016.09.013
22. Kozhimannil, K. B., Graves, A. J., Jarlenski, M., Kennedy-Hendricks, A., Gollust, S., & Barry, C. L. (2017). Non-medical opioid use and sources of opioids among pregnant and non-pregnant reproductive-aged women. *Drug and Alcohol Dependence, 174*, 201–208. https://doi.org/10.1016/j.drugalcdep.2017.01.003
23. Rose-Jacobs, R., Trevino-Talbot, M., Vibbert, M., Lloyd-Travaglini, C., & Cabral, H. J. (2019). Pregnant women in treatment for opioid use disorder: Material hardships and psychosocial factors. *Addictive Behaviors, 98*, 106030. https://doi.org/10.1016/j.addbeh.2019.106030
24. NTI Upstream (n.d.). *The 4P's Plus© screening instrument.* www.ntiupstream.com/4psabout
25. Trocin, K. E., Weinstein, N. I., Oga, E. A., Mark, K. S., & Coleman-Cowger, V. H. (2020). Prenatal practice staff perceptions of three substance use screening tools for pregnant women. *Journal of Addiction Medicine, 14*(2), 139–144. https://doi.org/10.1097/ADM.0000000000000543

26. Desrosiers, A., Thompson, A., Divney, A., Magriples, U., & Kershaw, T. (2016). Romantic partner influences on prenatal and postnatal substance use in young couples. *Journal of Public Health, 38*(2), 300–307. https://doi.org/10.1093/pubmed/fdv039
27. Asta, D., Davis, A., Krishnamurti, T., Klocke, L., Abdullah, W., & Krans, E. E. (2021). The influence of social relationships on substance use behaviors among pregnant women with opioid use disorder. *Drug and Alcohol Dependence, 222*, 108665. https://doi.org/10.1016/j.drugalcdep.2021.108665
28. Mian, M. N., Foti, T. R., Green, A., Iturralde, E., Altschuler, A., Does, M. B., Jackson-Morris, M., Adams, S. R., Satre, D. D., Ansley, D., & Young-Wolff, K. C. (2023). Exploring preferences for different modes of cannabis use during early pregnancy: A qualitative study. *Addictive Behaviors, 146*, 107812. https://doi.org/10.1016/j.addbeh.2023.107812
29. Voutilainen, T., Rysä, J., Keski-Nisula, L., & Kärkkäinen, O. (2022). Self-reported alcohol consumption of pregnant women and their partners correlates both before and during pregnancy: A cohort study with 21,472 singleton pregnancies. *Alcoholism, Clinical and Experimental Research, 46*(5), 797–808. https://doi.org/10.1111/acer.14806
30. Puurunen, K., & Vis, J. A. (2019). Pregnancy as an opportunity for trauma-intervention among women who are addicted to substances. *Journal of Aggression, Maltreatment & Trauma, 28*(3), 281–296. https://doi.org/10.1080/10926771.2017.1332703
31. Duka, S., Rahman, S., Hansen, S. E., & Esernio-Jenssen, D. (2023). The effect of maternal Adverse Childhood Experiences (ACEs) on substance use during pregnancy. *Maternal and Child Health Journal, 27*(Suppl 1), 153–165. https://doi.org/10.1007/s10995-023-03768-4
32. Miller-Graff, L. E., Howell, K. H., Grein, K., & Keough, K. (2021). Women's cigarette and marijuana use in pregnancy: Identifying the role of past versus recent violence exposure. *Journal of Interpersonal Violence, 36*(7–8). https://doi.org/10.1177/0886260518779068
33. Washio, Y., Mericle, A. A., Cassey, H., Daubert, A. M., & Kirby, K. C. (2016). Characteristics of low-income racial/ethnic minority pregnant women screening positive for alcohol risk. *Journal of Immigrant and Minority Health, 18*(4), 850–855. https://doi.org/10.1007/s10903-015-0238-5
34. O'Connor, M., Czarnik, M., Morrow, B., & D'Angelo, D. (2022). Opioid use during pregnancy: An analysis of comment data from the 2016 pregnancy risk assessment monitoring system survey. *Substance Abuse, 43*(1), 649–656. https://doi.org/10.1080/08897077.2021.1986878
35. Kotelchuck, M., Cheng, E. R., Belanoff, C., Cabral, H. J., Babakhanlou-Chase, H., Derrington, T. M., Diop, H., Evans, S. R., & Bernstein, J. (2017). The prevalence and impact of substance use disorder and treatment on maternal obstetric experiences and birth outcomes among singleton deliveries in Massachusetts. *Maternal and Child Health Journal, 21*(4), 893–902. https://doi.org/10.1007/s10995-016-2190-y
36. McCartin, M., Cannon, L. M., Harfmann, R. F., Dalton, V. K., MacAfee, L. K., & Kusunoki, Y. (2022). Stigma and reproductive health service access among women in treatment for substance use disorder. *Women's Health Issues, 32*(6), 595–601. https://doi.org/10.1016/j.whi.2022.06.003
37. Salameh, T. N., Hall, L. A., Crawford, T. N., Staten, R. R., & Hall, M. T. (2021). Likelihood of mental health and substance use treatment receipt among pregnant women in the USA. *International Journal of Mental Health and Addiction, 19*(5), 1569–1585. https://doi.org/10.1007/s11469-020-00247-7
38. Kramlich, D., Kronk, R., Marcellus, L., Colbert, A., & Jakub, K. (2018). Rural postpartum women with substance use disorders. *Qualitative Health Research, 28*(9), 1449–1461. https://doi.org/10.1177/1049732318765720
39. Qato, D. M., Zhang, C., Gandhi, A. B., Simoni-Wastila, L., & Coleman-Cowger, V. H. (2020). Co-use of alcohol, tobacco, and licit and illicit controlled substances among pregnant and non-pregnant women in the United States: Findings from 2006 to 2014 National Survey on Drug Use and Health (NSDUH) data. *Drug and Alcohol Dependence, 206*, 107729. https://doi.org/10.1016/j.drugalcdep.2019.107729
40. Board, A., D'Angelo, D. V., von Essen, B. S., Denny, C. H., Miele, K., Dunkley, J., Park, Y., & Kim, S. Y. (2023). The postpartum period: An opportunity for alcohol screening and counseling to reduce adverse health impacts. *Journal of Addiction Medicine, 17*(5), 528–535. https://doi.org/10.1097/ADM.0000000000001169

41. Smith, B. L., Hall, E. S., McAllister, J. M., Marcotte, M. P., Setchell, K. D. R., Megaraj, V., Jimenez, K. L., Winhusen, T. J., & Wexelblatt, S. L. (2022). Rates of substance and polysubstance use through universal maternal testing at the time of delivery. *Journal of Perinatology*, *42*(8), 1026–1031. https://doi.org/10.1038/s41372-022-01335-3
42. Hoffman, J. (2024, June). Pregnant, addicted, and fighting the pull of drugs. *The New York Times*. www.nytimes.com/2024/06/16/health/pregnancy-drug-addiction.html
43. U.S. Department of Health and Human Services (n.d.). *National opioids crisis: Help and resources*. www.hhs.gov/opioids/index.html. Accessed December 2024.
44. John Hopkins Medicine (n.d.). *Opioid use disorder*. www.hopkinsmedicine.org/health/conditions-and-diseases/opioid-use-disorder
45. Admon, L. K., Bart, G., Kozhimannil, K. B., Richardson, C. R., Dalton, V. K., & Winkelman, T. N. (2019). Amphetamine-and opioid-affected births: Incidence, outcomes, and costs, United States, 2004–2015. *American Journal of Public Health*, *109*(1), 148–154. https://doi.org/10.2105/AJPH.2018.304771
46. Ko, J. Y., D'Angelo, D. V., Haight, S. C., Morrow, B., Cox, S., Salvesen von Essen, B., Strahan, A., Harrison, L., Tevendale, H. D., Warner, L., Kroelinger, C. D., & Barfield, W. D. (2019). Vital signs: Prescription opioid pain reliever use during pregnancy – 34 U.S. jurisdictions. *Morbidity and Mortality Weekly Report*, *69*, 897–903. https://doi.org/10.15585/mmwr.mm6928a1. Accessed December 2024.
47. Han, B., Compton, W. M., Einstein, E. B., Elder, E., & Volkow, N. D. (2024). Pregnancy and postpartum drug overdose deaths in the US before and during the COVID-19 pandemic. *JAMA Psychiatry*, *81*(3), 270–283. https://doi.org/10.1001/jamapsychiatry.2023.4523
48. Horn, A., Adgent, M. A., Osmundson, S. S., Wiese, A. D., Phillips, S. E., Patrick, S. W., Griffin, M. R., & Grijalva, C. G. (2024). Risk of death at 1 year following postpartum opioid exposure. *American Journal of Perinatology*, *41*(7), 949–960. https://doi.org/10.1055/s-0042-1745848
49. Powell, D. (2023). Educational attainment and US drug overdose deaths. *JAMA Health Forum*, *4*(10), e233274. https://doi.org/10.1001/jamahealthforum.2023.3274
50. Daniels, S., St Pierre, M., Sanchez, T., & Walsh, Z. (2023). Physician communication and perceived stigma in prenatal cannabis use. *Journal of Psychoactive Drugs*, *55*(3), 290–298. https://doi.org/10.1080/02791072.2022.2076179
51. Shen, Y., Lo-Ciganic, W. H., Segal, R., & Goodin, A. J. (2020). Prevalence of substance use disorder and psychiatric comorbidity burden among pregnant women with opioid use disorder in a large administrative database, 2009–2014. *Journal of Psychosomatic Obstetrics and Gynaecology*, 1–7. https://doi.org/10.1080/0167482X.2020.1727882
52. Testa, A., Crawford, A. D., Jackson, D. B., & Gemmill, A. (2022). Stressful life events and prescription opioid use during pregnancy: Findings from the 2019 pregnancy risk assessment monitoring system. *Social Psychiatry and Psychiatric Epidemiology*, *57*(11), 2181–2191. https://doi.org/10.1007/s00127-022-02349-0
53. Rankin, L., Mendoza, N. S., & Grisham, L. (2023). Unpacking perinatal experiences with opioid use disorder: Relapse risk implications. *Clinical Social Work Journal*, *51*(1), 34–45. https://doi.org/10.1007/s10615-022-00847-x
54. National Institute on Drug Abuse (2017, May). *Medications to treat opioid disorder research report: What treatment is available for pregnant mothers and their babies*? https://nida.nih.gov/publications/research-reports/medications-to-treat-opioid-addiction/what-treatment-available-pregnant-mothers-their-babies#:~:text=To%20lessen%20the%20negative%20effects,standard%20of%20care%20since%201998.&text=Recent%20evidence%2C%20however%2C%20suggests%20that,an%20even%20better%20treatment%20option. Accessed December 2024.
55. Carley, J. A., & Oesterle, T. (2021). Therapeutic approaches to opioid use disorder: What is the current standard of care? *International Journal of General Medicine*, *14*, 2305–2311. https://doi.org/10.2147/IJGM.S295461
56. Mette, E., Manz, J., Purington, K., & Antezzo, M. (2021). *State approaches to leveraging neonatal abstinence syndrome data to inform policymaking*. https://nashp.org/state-approaches-to-leveraging-neonatal-abstinence-syndrome-data-to-inform-policymaking/#:~:text=Under%20CAPTA%2FCARA%2C%20states%20must,infant%20and%20the%20parent%20or

57. Casey Family Programs (2024). *Plans of safe care.* www.casey.org/infant-plans-of-safe-care/.
58. National Harm Reduction Coalition (n.d.). *Opioid overdose basics: Recognizing opioid overdose.* https://harmreduction.org/issues/overdose-prevention/overview/overdose-basics/recognizing-opioid-overdose/
59. The American College of Obstetricians and Gynecologists (2017, October). *Marijuana use during pregnancy and lactation.* www.acog.org/clinical/clinical-guidance/committee-opinion/articles/2017/10/marijuana-use-during-pregnancy-and-lactation
60. Ryan, K. S., Bash, J. C., Hanna, C. B., Hedges, J. C., & Lo, J. O. (2021). Effects of marijuana on reproductive health: Preconception and gestational effects. *Current Opinion in Endocrinology, Diabetes, and Obesity, 28*(6), 558–565. https://doi.org/10.1097/MED.0000000000000686
61. U.S. Centers for Disease Control and Prevention (n.d.). *Cannabis and pregnancy.* www.cdc.gov/cannabis/health-effects/pregnancy.html
62. March of Dimes (2020, September). *Marijuana and pregnancy.* www.marchofdimes.org/find-support/topics/pregnancy/marijuana-and-pregnancy
63. Shi, Y., Zhu, B., & Liang, D. (2021). The associations between prenatal cannabis use disorder and neonatal outcomes. *Addiction, 116*(11), 3069–3079. https://doi.org/10.1111/add.15467
64. McKenzie, L. B., Keim, S. A., & Klebanoff, M. A. (2022). Risk perceptions about cannabis use and receipt of health-related information during pregnancy. *American Journal of Health Promotion, 36*(8), 1316–1325. https://doi.org/10.1177/08901171221099496
65. Alshaarawy, O., & Vanderziel, A. (2022). Trends and characteristics of prenatal cannabis use in the U.S., 2002–2019. *American Journal of Preventive Medicine, 63*(5), 846–851. https://doi.org/10.1016/j.amepre.2022.04.027
66. Young-Wolff, K. C., Sarovar, V., Tucker, L. Y., Ansley, D., Goler, N., Conway, A., Ettenger, A., Foti, T. R., Brown, Q. L., Kurtzman, E. T., Adams, S. R., & Alexeeff, S. E. (2022). Trends in cannabis polysubstance use during early pregnancy among patients in a large health care system in Northern California. *JAMA Network Open, 5*(6), e2215418. https://doi.org/10.1001/jamanetworkopen.2022.15418
67. Badowski, S., & Smith, G. (2020). Cannabis use during pregnancy and postpartum. *Canadian Family Physician, 66*(2), 98–103.
68. Ko, J. Y., Coy, K. C., Haight, S. C., Haegerich, T. M., Williams, L., Cox, S., Njai, R., & Grant, A. M. (2020). Characteristics of marijuana use during pregnancy – Eight states, pregnancy risk assessment monitoring system, 2017. *Morbidity and Mortality Weekly Report, 69*, 1058–1063. https://doi.org/10.15585/mmwr.mm6932a2. Accessed December 2024.
69. Alexander, M. (2010). *The new Jim Crow: Mass incarceration in the age of colorblindness.* The New Press.
70. Green, P. P., McKnight-Eily, L. R., Tan, C. H., Mejia, R., & Denny, C. H. (2016). Vital signs: Alcohol-exposed pregnancies – United States, 2011–2013. *Morbidity and Mortality Weekly Report, 65*(4), 91–97. https://doi.org/10.15585/mmwr.mm6504a6. Accessed December 2024.
71. Phillips, D. P., Brewer, K. M., & Wadensweiler, P. (2011). Alcohol as a risk factor for sudden infant death syndrome (SIDS). *Addiction, 106*(3), 516–525. https://doi.org/10.1111/j.1360-0443.2010.03199.x
72. The American College of Obstetricians and Gynecologists (2024). *Alcohol and pregnancy.* www.acog.org/womens-health/infographics/alcohol-and-pregnancy#:~:text=Didn't%20know%20you%20were,find%20out%20you%20are%20pregnant
73. Adiri, C. O., Asimadu, E. E., Nwafor, M. I., Nweze, S. O., & Ukaegbe, C. I. (2022). Perception of safety and consumption of alcoholic beverages during pregnancy. *Journal of Obstetrics and Gynaecology, 42*(7), 3021–3025. https://doi.org/10.1080/01443615.2022.2125795
74. Sundermann, A. C., Velez Edwards, D. R., Slaughter, J. C., Wu, P., Jones, S. H., Torstenson, E. S., & Hartmann, K. E. (2021). Week-by-week alcohol consumption in early pregnancy and spontaneous abortion risk: A prospective cohort study. *American Journal of Obstetrics and Gynecology, 224*(1), 97.e1–97.e16. https://doi.org/10.1016/j.ajog.2020.07.012
75. Canver, B. R., Newman, R. K., & Gomez, A. E. (2024, January). *Alcohol withdrawal syndrome.* StatPearls Publishing. www.ncbi.nlm.nih.gov/books/NBK441882/
76. Chapman, M., Bandoli, G., & Goldenberg, S. M. (2024). The association between depression and alcohol use among pregnant adults in the USA. *Archives of Women's Mental Health, 27*(3), 425–433. https://doi.org/10.1007/s00737-023-01417-x

77. Sundermann, A. C., Velez Edwards, D. R., Slaughter, J. C., Wu, P., Jones, S. H., Torstenson, E. S., & Hartmann, K. E. (2021). Week-by-week alcohol consumption in early pregnancy and spontaneous abortion risk: A prospective cohort study. *American Journal of Obstetrics and Gynecology, 224*(1), 97.e1–97.e16. https://doi.org/10.1016/j.ajog.2020.07.012
78. Board, A., D'Angelo, D. V., Salvesen von Essen, B., Denny, C. H., Miele, K., Dunkley, J., Baillieu, R., & Kim, S. Y. (2023). Polysubstance use during pregnancy: The importance of screening, patient education, and integrating a harm reduction perspective. *Drug and Alcohol Dependence, 247*, 109872. https://doi.org/10.1016/j.drugalcdep.2023.109872
79. Laborde, N. D., & Mair, C. (2012). Alcohol use patterns among postpartum women. *Maternal and Child Health Journal, 16*(9), 1810–1819. https://doi.org/10.1007/s10995-011-0925-3
80. U.S. Centers for Disease Control and Prevention (n.d.). *Breastfeeding special circumstances: Alcohol.* www.cdc.gov/breastfeeding-special-circumstances/hcp/vaccine-medication-drugs/alcohol.html. Accessed December 2024.
81. Marufu, T. C., Ahankari, A., Coleman, T., & Lewis, S. (2015). Maternal smoking and the risk of still birth: Systematic review and meta-analysis. *BMC Public Health, 15*(1), 1–15. https://doi.org/10.1186/s12889-015-1552-5
82. Kipling, L., Bombard, J., Wang, X., & Cox, S. (2021). Cigarette smoking among pregnant women during the perinatal period: Prevalence and health care provider inquiries – Pregnancy Risk Assessment Monitoring System, United States, 2021. *Morbidity and Mortality Weekly Report, 73*, 393–398. https://doi.org/10.15585/mmwr.mm7317a2. Accessed December 2024.
83. The American College of Obstetricians and Gynecologists (2020, May). *Tobacco and nicotine cessation during pregnancy.* www.acog.org/clinical/clinical-guidance/committee-opinion/articles/2020/05/tobacco-and-nicotine-cessation-during-pregnancy
84. Shobeiri, F., & Jenabi, E. (2017). Smoking and placenta previa: A meta-analysis. *The Journal of Maternal-Fetal & Neonatal Medicine, 30*(24), 2985–2990. https://doi.org/10.1080/14767058.2016.1271405
85. Wei, J., Liu, C. X., Gong, T. T., Wu, Q. J., & Wu, L. (2015). Cigarette smoking during pregnancy and preeclampsia risk: A systematic review and meta-analysis of prospective studies. *Oncotarget, 6*(41), 43667. https://doi.org/10.18632/oncotarget.6190
86. Ezegbe, C., Neil, A. L., Magnussen, C. G., Chappell, K., Judd, F., Wagg, F., & Gall, S. (2021). Maternal smoking during pregnancy: Trends and determinants in the conception to community study. *Birth, 48*(1), 76–85. https://doi.org/10.1111/birt.12515
87. Vilcassim, M. J. R., Stowe, S., Majumder, R., Subramaniam, A., & Sinkey, R. G. (2023). Electronic cigarette use during pregnancy: Is it harmful? *Toxics, 11*(3), 278. https://doi.org/10.3390/toxics11030278
88. Wen, X., Liu, L., Moe, A. A., Ormond, I. K., Shuren, C. C., Scott, I. N., Ozga, J. E., Stanton, C. A., Ruybal, A. L., Hart, J. L., Goniewicz, M. L., Lee, D., & Vargees, C. (2023). Use of e-cigarettes and cigarettes during late pregnancy among adolescents. *JAMA Network Open, 6*(12), e2347407. https://doi.org/10.1001/jamanetworkopen.2023.47407
89. Blatt, K., Moore, E., Chen, A., Van Hook, J., & DeFranco, E. A. (2015). Association of reported trimester-specific smoking cessation and fetal growth restriction. *Obstetrics and Gynecology, 125*(6), 1452. https://doi.org/10.1097/AOG.0000000000000679
90. Wilson, S. M., Newins, A. R., Medenblik, A. M., Kimbrel, N. A., Dedert, E. A., Hicks, T. A., Neal, L. C., Beckham, J. C., & Calhoun, P. S. (2018). Contingency management versus psychotherapy for prenatal smoking cessation: A meta-analysis of randomized controlled trials. *Women's Health Issues, 28*(6), 514–523. https://doi.org/10.1016/j.whi.2018.05.002
91. Shisler, S., Homish, G. G., Molnar, D. S., Schuetze, P., Colder, C. R., & Eiden, R. D. (2016). Predictors of changes in smoking from third trimester to 9 months postpartum. *Nicotine & Tobacco Research, 18*(1), 84–87. https://doi.org/10.1093/ntr/ntv057
92. Wen, K. Y., Miller, S. M., Roussi, P., Belton, T. D., Baman, J., Kilby, L., & Hernandez, E. (2015). A content analysis of self-reported barriers and facilitators to preventing postpartum smoking relapse among a sample of current and former smokers in an underserved population. *Health Education Research, 30*(1), 140–151. https://doi.org/10.1093/her/cyu048
93. Singhal, N., Fauth, R. C., Thompson, M., Posner, E., & Moosmann, D. A. V. (2023). *Recovery support through home visiting.* Tufts Interdisciplinary Evaluation Research (TIER). Tufts University.

5 Death During Pregnancy, the Postpartum Period, and the First Year of Life

Self-Care Moment

Death can be an especially difficult topic to read about, particularly if you have experienced loss or grief in your own life. Before continuing with this chapter, take a minute to do something soothing for your body or mind – for example, standing up to stretch, getting a cup of tea, or texting a friend. Also consider how you will take care of yourself during and after reading this chapter – for example, doing deep breathing or sensory grounding, taking breaks, or planning a relaxing activity for later today.

Death during pregnancy, the postpartum period, and the first year of life (including miscarriage and stillbirth) is much less common in the twenty-first century than it was in the past (though still much more common than it should be, given advances in knowledge and medicine). Still, every loss is a tragedy. These deaths have tremendous impacts on families and communities, sometimes for years or generations to come.

Tragically, research has also shown that most deaths during pregnancy, the postpartum period, and the first year of life could have been prevented with earlier or more appropriate intervention, and that some groups (i.e., people of color, people experiencing poverty) are less likely to receive such interventions and are thus more likely to die. Furthermore, while the media often publicize tragedies that occur during active labor and delivery, the reality is that the highest number of deaths occur during pregnancy and the postpartum period (days or even weeks after childbirth). Thus, this chapter focuses on risk and protective factors for death during these periods, including a discussion of research on this topic, practice implications for your work, and reflections on your role as a community or social service provider. You will also hear the stories of two women who tragically died from complications related to pregnancy and childbirth, Amber Rose Isaac and Tori Bowie, and the story of a home visiting program that introduced a safe sleep initiative for families with infants.

Amber's Story ∞

Amber Rose Isaac's fiancé Bruce remembers her as "an inspiration to many, a leader among her peers, and an innovator who was going to shape the world in one way or another."[1]

DOI: 10.4324/9781003476474-5

Amber, a 26-year-old Black Puerto Rican woman from New York, tragically died in 2020 from complications related to HELLP syndrome following an emergency C-section.[2] HELLP is a group of symptoms that includes **H**emolysis (breakdown of red blood cells), **E**levated **L**iver enzymes, and **L**ow **P**latelet count. Throughout her pregnancy, Amber had shared concerns about numerous health symptoms with her doctors – for example, her platelet levels, dizziness, headaches, chest pain, and shortness of breath – only to be dismissed. On social media, she expressed frustration with the quality of care that she was receiving. Heartbreakingly, many of the symptoms that Amber was trying to draw attention to were signs of the HELLP syndrome that ultimately took her life. In subsequent interviews and testimonies, Bruce has recalled how, from the start of Amber's pregnancy until her death, her medical care was characterized by biases and errors – leaving him without his life partner, and their newborn son Elias without his mother.[1,2]

Tori's Story ∞

Several years later, in 2023, the tragic death of 32-year-old Olympic sprinter Tori Bowie brought international attention to the realities of maternal death.[3] Tori, a Black woman, died alone in her Florida home while in active labor at eight months pregnant. Her baby also died. An autopsy cited complications from eclampsia, high blood pressure, and respiratory distress. Tori's loved ones and neighbors also shared that her pregnancy had been difficult, that she was struggling with bipolar disorder, and that her behavior had markedly changed shortly before her death. Tori's heartbreaking death reflects not only the dangers of preeclampsia, but the persistent failures in identifying and addressing physical and mental health needs during pregnancy. Her story is part of a broader crisis that disproportionately impacts Black women, who are significantly more likely to die during pregnancy, childbirth, and the postpartum period than their White counterparts in the United States.

Research Summary

Death During Pregnancy and the Postpartum Period

Rates and Disparities

Death rates during pregnancy and the postpartum period have risen over the past 20 years in the United States and have doubled since the year 2000 – statistics which are partially related to better reporting, but also to many inequities and disparities.[4,5] In a recent report on maternal deaths in the United States, the maternal death rate was reported in the year 2022 at 22.3 deaths per 100,000 live births.[6] Notably, a 2017–2019 review of data from maternal mortality review committees across the United States determined that 80% of pregnancy-related deaths were due to preventable causes.[7]

Racial and ethnic disparities are strongly evident in maternal death rates in the United States and beyond, with the National Center for Health Statistics reporting wide gaps in death rates between non-Hispanic Black, non-Hispanic White, and Hispanic women (49.5, 19.0, and 16.9 deaths per 100,000 live births, respectively).[6] Across studies, the racial disparity between non-Hispanic Black women and White women tends to be most prominent, even after accounting for factors that tend to be protective against negative health outcomes.[8,9,10,11] One study indicated that while White mothers were less likely to die if they had higher levels of education, there was minimal difference in death rates for Black mothers with a college degree versus Black mothers with less than a high school education.[12] The same research further showed that maternal deaths were more common among Black mothers with a college education than among White mothers with less than a high school education.

Similar disparities are found in Indigenous populations. Research has documented elevated death rates among Indigenous mothers in the United States, particularly those living in rural areas, compared to White mothers.[13,14,15] Taken together, these findings point to the deep role that systemic racism plays in shaping health outcomes. Disparities in death rates have also been reported between people with different types of insurance coverage. One study reported that Black women, as well as mothers with public insurance coverage, often believe that their healthcare providers did not respect them or empower them to make decisions during childbirth.[16] These and other findings highlight the importance of considering how structural bias and racism can impact experiences within healthcare systems during pregnancy and the postpartum period.[17]

Timing and Causes

National data in the United States has revealed that the most frequent causes of pregnancy-related death are mental health conditions (see Chapters 3–4 for more detailed discussion of these conditions), hemorrhage (severe bleeding), cardiac (heart) and coronary conditions, and infection.[7] It is believed that more than 80% of these deaths could have been prevented with timely and effective intervention.[7]

Take Time to Reflect

Read the preceding paragraph again. What emotions, physical sensations, or thoughts do you notice when reading that more than 80% of pregnancy-related deaths in the United States could have been prevented? Consider what you have heard about maternal death. How has it impacted your community? How frequently is it talked about? How might you get to know more about the state of maternal death in your community?

Tragically, suicide is a leading cause of death for pregnant and postpartum individuals, and they are also at increased risk for death by homicide – with about five homicides occurring out of every 100,000 individuals who give birth to a live infant in the United St ates.[18,19,20,21] These statistics underscore a critical need for policies and interventions that increase access to mental health and social services, and reduce rates of community and intimate partner violence.

Individuals struggling with substance misuse are also at increased risk of death during pregnancy and the postpartum period. One large multi-year study in the United States indicated that those with opioid use disorder were six times more likely to die in the first year after giving birth, compared to postpartum individuals without opioid use disorder. Common causes include opioid overdose, non-opioid substance-related injuries, accidents, and suicide.[22]

Leading causes of death during pregnancy and the postpartum period vary by race and ethnicity, highlighting disparities in SDOH and access to intervention. For example, data from the U.S. National Center for Health Statistics revealed that cardiovascular (heart) conditions, hemorrhage, and hypertensive disorders were more common causes of death among people of color than their White counterparts, with further differences detected among non-Hispanic Black, Hispanic, and Indigenous groups.[23] Another study reported that the leading causes of death were: (a) cardiovascular conditions for Black (non-Hispanic) individuals; (b) mental health conditions for Hispanic and non-Hispanic White individuals; and (c) hemorrhage for Asian (non-Hispanic) individuals. The same study demonstrated additional patterns in causes of death based on age, body mass index (BMI), and method of delivery.[23]

The media often publicize tragedies that occur during labor and delivery. However, in the United States, over half of maternal deaths occur during the postpartum period, and about one-third occur outside of a medical facility.[16,24] Between 2017 and 2019, pregnancy-related deaths in the United States were most likely to occur 43–365 days postpartum (30% of deaths), followed by 7–42 days postpartum (23.3%) and during pregnancy (21.6%). A smaller number of deaths occurred on the day of delivery (13.2%) and within between one and six days of giving birth (12.0%).[7]

Research has also shown that the leading causes of pregnancy-related death vary based on the timepoint at which they occur (pregnancy, labor and delivery, postpartum period). Table 5.1 describes the timing of leading causes of pregnancy-related death in the United States based on national datasets.[23,25]

Table 5.1 Timing and Causes of Pregnancy-Related Deaths in the United States

Timing and Causes of Pregnancy-Related Deaths, 2011–2015
Source: United States Pregnancy Mortality Surveillance System[13]

Cause of Death	*Most Common Time (% of Deaths Due to That Cause)*	*Second-Most Common Time (% of Deaths Due to That Cause)*	*Third-Most Common Time (% of Deaths Due to That Cause)*	*% of All Deaths (Out of 2,990 Deaths)*
Thrombotic pulmonary or other embolism	During pregnancy (40.9%)	Seven to 42 days postpartum (24.6%)	One to six days postpartum (14.6%)	9.4%
Other cardiovascular conditions	During pregnancy (37.6%)	Seven to 42 days postpartum (23.9%)	Day of delivery (14.1%)	15.4%
Other non-cardiovascular medical conditions	During pregnancy (52.7%)	Day of delivery (14.3%)	Seven to 42 days of delivery (13.8%)	14.3%
Unknown causes	During pregnancy (40.4%)	Seven to 42 days postpartum (24.6%)	Day of delivery (13.8%)	6.8%
Hemorrhage	Day of delivery (37.4%)	One to six days postpartum (31.9%)	During pregnancy (21.9%)	11.0%
Amniotic fluid embolism	Day of delivery (65.9%)	One to six days postpartum (24.3%)	During pregnancy (6.9%)	5.7%

(*Continued*)

Table 5.1 (Continued)

Timing and Causes of Pregnancy-Related Deaths, 2011–2015
Source: United States Pregnancy Mortality Surveillance System

Cause of Death	*Most Common Time (% of Deaths Due to That Cause)*	*Second-Most Common Time (% of Deaths Due to That Cause)*	*Third-Most Common Time (% of Deaths Due to That Cause)*	*% of All Deaths (Out of 2,990 Deaths)*
Anesthesia complications	Day of delivery (30.0%) and 1–6 days postpartum (30.0%)	–	Seven to 42 days postpartum (20.0%) and during pregnancy (20.0%)	0.3%
Hypertensive disorders of pregnancy	One to six days postpartum (44.3%)	Seven to 42 days postpartum (20.8%)	Day of delivery (19.3%)	7.1%
Infection	Seven to 42 days postpartum (33.6%)	During pregnancy (32.5%)	One to six days postpartum (23.1%)	12.0%
Cerebrovascular accidents	Seven to 42 days postpartum (34.6%)	During pregnancy (29.8%)	One to six days postpartum (21.5%)	7.6%
Cardiomyopathy	Forty-three to 365 days postpartum (45.0%)	Seven to 42 days postpartum (24.4%)	During pregnancy (15.6%)	10.3%
Suicide and "deaths of undetermined intent"	Forty-three to 365 days postpartum (42.7%)	During pregnancy (39.6%)	One to 42 days postpartum (17.7%)	–

Take Time to Reflect

In the United States, maternal death is most likely to occur a week or more after giving birth. What implications might this have for the education or follow-up that you provide within your role as a community or social service provider?

Risk and Protective Factors

Certain experiences and factors can increase the risk of maternal death, such as chronic illness (i.e., Type 2 diabetes, asthma), lifestyle factors (i.e., pre-pregnancy weight, nutrition, physical activity), and living in a "maternity care desert" (i.e., a region where there are no nearby hospitals or providers that offer obstetric care).[26,27] All these factors are closely linked to SDOH (i.e., education access and quality, healthcare access and quality, neighborhood and built environment, social and community context, economic stability).[28]

Another study indicated that when pregnant and postpartum individuals have low health literacy, there is an increased risk of death.[29] For example, research has found that many new mothers are not aware of all the key warning signs or complications that can arise during the postpartum period, or the steps that they should take if they experience them.[30] These findings highlight the importance of providing health education throughout pregnancy and the postpartum period in language which is easy to understand.

Access to preconception healthcare and family planning supports, and a full range of healthcare supports from the beginning to the end of pregnancy (see Chapters 6–8 for further discussion), are also important strategies for preventing maternal death. Barriers to these services, such as legal restrictions, stigma, and cost can make it difficult for people to access the care that they need and, in some cases, increase the risk of de ath.[31,32,33,34]

Putting It Into Practice

- ***Discuss family planning as a standard part of services with all families.*** Keep in mind that very short (less than six months) or very long (60–100 months) intervals between the end of one pregnancy and the start of another carry risks for both maternal and infant health. Initiate conversations about family planning by acknowledging that this is a personal topic, while also providing clear rationale for why it is important to discuss. Help parents to reflect on their values and goals and encourage them to talk to their healthcare provider about any family planning needs. Increasingly, it is also important for all providers to keep up to date with local options related to preconception healthcare, family planning, contraception, pregnancy and postpartum care.
- ***Provide timely information about physical and social/emotional changes during pregnancy and the postpartum period, including key warning signs or complications for which to watch.*** As discussed in Chapter 3, many people do not know the warning signs of serious physical or mental health challenges during pregnancy and the postpartum period, or what to do if problems arise. Healthcare providers may not explain this information in easy-to-understand ways, and for some families, there may also be language or other factors that affect their understanding of the information provided. Reinforce and build on information that your clients and members of their support systems may (or may not) have heard in healthcare visits. Community and social service providers often have more time to have in-depth conversations with families than healthcare providers. The trusting relationships built between community and social service providers and the families they serve can create spaces for asking questions and reflecting on information and advice they have received from different sources (i.e., their healthcare provider, family members,).
- ***Make and assist with resource connections.*** You can support clients in navigating complex healthcare and social service systems, including medical care, mental healthcare, intimate partner violence resources, housing, food resources, and more. Supporting clients on these fronts can be especially impactful during and after pregnancy. Key resources that can be especially protective against infant death include having health insurance and maternal/child health or social services (such as the Women, Infants, and Children [WIC] program in the United States). It is often most efficient and effective to connect families to these resources when your programs have written cooperative agreements with each other. Work with

your program leaders and colleagues to build a network of services to which you can more easily connect families.

- ***Support healthcare advocacy.*** Support your pregnant and postpartum clients (and their family members) in formulating questions about their health and healthcare options, and to make plans for how they will reach out to their healthcare providers when questions or concerns arise. Reaching out can be especially challenging for individuals whose healthcare providers previously dismissed their concerns. In these situations, practice or role-play with your clients and their family members to build their confidence before they interact with a healthcare provider. In some cases, it may be helpful to facilitate connections with a doula or other healthcare advocate who can attend medical appointments and perhaps even childbirth.
- ***Plan to touch base with families in the days following delivery.*** The first days at home following a birth can be emotional and stressful, on top of the experience of physically recovering from giving birth. Even before they give birth, you can discuss your anticipated availability following the delivery. You can set up planned times to connect but also make clear that they can reach out to you with concerns. As reflected in Cam's story from Chapter 2, validating concerns and encouraging follow-up can be life-saving.

Death Among Infants

Key Terms

Miscarriage: Loss of a fetus or baby relatively early in pregnancy. In the United States, losses are considered miscarriages if they occur at 20 weeks gestation or earlier.[35] In other parts of the world, losses are considered miscarriages up to 28 weeks gestation.[36]

Stillbirth: Loss of a fetus or baby late in pregnancy or at labor or delivery. In the United States, losses are considered stillbirths if they occur after 20 weeks gestation.[35] In other parts of the world, losses are considered stillbirths if they occur after 28 weeks gestation.[36]

Infant mortality: Death of a baby occurring after birth, up until the first birthday.

Neonatal mortality: Death of an infant occurring between zero and 27 days after birth.[37]

Postnatal mortality: Death of an infant occurring between 28 and 364 days after birth.[37]

Sudden unexpected infant death (SUID): Any sudden, unexpected infant death. This category includes deaths from unknown causes as well as deaths from known causes (i.e., accidents or injuries, including those related to how or where a baby sleeps).

Sudden infant death syndrome (SIDS): A sudden, unexpected infant death with no known causes, even after a full medical examination.

Infant/child maltreatment: Abuse or neglect, including but not limited to physical, emotional, and sexual abuse; neglect and negligence; and exploitation.

Infant mortality rate: In the United States, the number of infants who die before their first birthday out of every 1,000 live births.
Inter-pregnancy interval: The amount of time between completing one pregnancy and starting another.

Rates and Disparities

Infant death rates follow many similar patterns as those described in the preceding key terms. The infant mortality rate (IMR) in the United States is among the highest of countries of similar economic status, with a rate of 5.6 infant deaths per 1,000 live births in 2022.[38]

Similar to disparities in maternal death, disparities in infant death rates have been identified related to race and ethnicity, particularly for Black, Native American, and Hispanic/Latinx infants.[37,39,40] These racial and ethnic disparities persist when comparing infants of color with college-educated parents to White infants with parents with high school educations or less.[41] Research has also shown links between racial disparities in infant death rates and racial inequities in several other domains. For example, racial inequities in education, work, home ownership, and other factors have been linked to higher death rates among Black infants in the United States. States with higher levels of income inequality also have higher infant and neonatal death rates.[42,43,44,45] One study indicated that growing racial inequity in unemployment was associated with a 5% increase in death rates among Black infants, while decreasing racial inequity in education was associated with an almost 10% reduction in death rates among Black infants.[46] At the local community level, research has shown that Black and Hispanic infants are more likely to be born in hospitals with historically elevated rates of infant health complications and death rates, further contributing to disparate outcomes.[47]

Timing and Causes

In the United States, the average number of deaths during the neonatal period (between zero and 27 days after birth) was about four (4) deaths for every 1,000 live births in 2022; during the postnatal period (between 28 and 364 days after birth) it was about two (2) deaths for every 1,000 live births. Leading causes of death for infants in the United States include birth defects, preterm birth and low birthweight, SIDS, accidental injuries, and maternal complications of pregnancy.[38] Across the United States and beyond, sleep-related SUID continue to be a leading cause of death among infants. Research has shown that despite widespread campaigns on safe sleep and risk reduction,[48] many infants still sleep in unsafe sleep conditions.[49,50,51] Researchers have found that sleep-related SUID most frequently occur when infants co-sleep or share a sleep surface with others, sleep on their stomach, are placed on a pillow, and/or have their heads covered with a blanket or other object.[52]

Take Action

Guidelines for safe sleep have evolved in recent years to reduce accidental sleep-related deaths. Take some time to refresh your understanding by opening a search engine and typing "safe sleep guidelines." Be sure to review websites and resources from reputable organizations, such as the American Academy of Pediatrics.

Risk and Protective Factors

Risks of and protections against infant death have been widely researched. One key risk factor is the time between completing one pregnancy and starting another, also known as the ***inter-pregnancy interval***. Research has shown that having an inter-pregnancy interval of less than six months is associated with increased risk of stillbirth, compared to pregnancies when the inter-pregnancy interval was 18–23 months. On the opposite end, longer inter-pregnancy intervals between 60 and 100 months have also been linked to negative pregnancy outcomes.[53] Research has also reported elevated rates of death among infants whose parents had lost previous pregnancies. One study reported that having three or more pregnancy losses or a loss within two years was associated with greater risk of negative pregnancy outcomes.[54] Another study indicated that individuals who had a stillbirth in their first pregnancy were five times more likely to experience a stillbirth in a second pregnancy.[55] Families who experience stillbirth need knowledgeable, sensitive psychosocial support that is individualized to their situation.[56,57]

Preterm birth is another known risk factor for infant death, which is often related to other health conditions or stressors. Most premature births are categorized as *late preterm* (between 34 weeks and 36 weeks and 6 days gestation). Late preterm infants have a greater risk of death than more mature infants and often require ongoing medical monitoring past the newborn period.[58]

Among infants who died from accidental injury (a leading cause of death among this age group), researchers have found that birth order and singleton versus multiple births are key factors. One study pulling from national data found that accidental injuries and other external causes of death were more likely between 2 and 7 months of age for multiples, such as twins and triplets.[59] Small inter-pregnancy interval is again a risk factor, with multiple studies linking shorter timing between births to higher rates of fatal injury among infants.[59,60] These findings are likely reflective of the increased stressors faced by parents with multiple children, particularly ones close in age.

Overall, differences in birth-related and/or sudden infant deaths are evident based on parental health, lifestyle factors, and education.[39,61,62,63] One study reported that risk for SUID more than doubled with any level of maternal smoking during pregnancy, and that nearly one-quarter of SUIDs in the United States could be directly attributed to smoking during pregnancy.[64] Other work has reported increased rates of stillbirth among people with pre-pregnancy obesity and/or gestational diabetes.[65,66]

Infants under the age of 1 year are also at heightened risk for maltreatment-related deaths compared to older children. In the United States, about three-quarters of maltreatment-related deaths involved neglect, and about 40% involved physical abuse (in some cases, both).[67] There are many risk and protective factors for infant maltreatment at the parent/caregiver, family, and community levels. Notably, higher rates of maltreatment have been found among parents and caregivers struggling with high levels of stress, mental health challenges, and/or substance use, whereas strong social support is a significant protective factor.[68]

Taken together, these findings highlight the importance of helping families to access the family planning, healthcare, parenting supports, and social services that they need during pregnancy and beyond.[69] Research has shown that benefits from public insurance coverage and social service programs protection offer some protection against infant death and related disparities. One study reported that in the United States, states that expanded access to public insurance saw greater reductions in infant death than states that did not expand access, and that these declines were greater among Black infants.[70] Other work has found that those with public insurance coverage and social service benefits during their pregnancy had lower likelihoods of infant death compared to those without insurance or social service coverage.[71]

Research has also pointed to the importance of facilitating culturally sensitive conversations with families and communities about infant death. In one interview-based study, Black participants reported that, in their experience, many community members tend to avoid the topic of infant death and see it as an unpreventable occurrence – despite the fact that community, social, and healthcare interventions can significantly reduce risk.[72]

The "Safe Sleep Project" at All for Kids' Home Visiting Program/ Infant and Toddler Home Visitation Δ

Many home visiting programs have implemented safe sleep initiatives to improve maternal and infant health and reduce the risk of SIDS. After receiving a grant, All for Kids' Home Visiting Program/Infant and Toddler Home Visitation in Southern California started a "Safe Sleep Project" that trains parent educators to perform safe sleep assessments during home visits and provide necessary education and resources to families. Following are several stories from the Safe Sleep Project.

> Sonia came to the United States from Guatemala less than two years ago and now rents a single room in a two-bedroom apartment. When Sonia's parent educator discovered that Sonia and her 7-month-old baby were sharing a bed and Sonia's husband, Francisco, was sleeping on the floor, they purchased the family a crib, safe sleep sacks, and pacifiers. The baby has been sleeping in the crib ever since, and Sonia and Francisco now have more restful nights of sleep with Sonia reporting, "I feel peaceful that my baby is safe in his crib, I like the crib very much! He will grow safe in his crib and this is a big crib that will last until he is a little older. I wanted to thank Parents as Teachers that provided the crib, because this was a great help for my child's safety, God bless you for all you do for my baby."
>
> Laura rents a room from family members and shares it with her 9-month-old daughter. During a safe sleep assessment, Laura's parent educator discovered that the baby had outgrown her bassinet as she was beginning to roll over and develop her gross motor skills. Laura had been sharing a bed with her daughter for some time out of fear that she could fall from the bassinet. The parent educator helped Laura purchase a new crib, mattress, and safe sleep sack for her child. Laura mentioned that having a safe sleeping space for her baby has given her peace of mind, and she continues to practice additional safe sleep behaviors discussed with her parent educator, such as laying the baby on her back and maintaining a clear sleep surface.
>
> One parent educator reported working with a first-time mother and father and their 2-month-old baby who all shared a bed with designated space against the wall for the baby to sleep due to the small size of the room they rent. The parent educator explained the dangers of co-sleeping and offered to purchase the family a bassinet for the baby. The bassinet did not take up much space in their room, and

the family reported having more restful nights and being grateful for the bassinet as well as the information provided on safe sleep practices.

During a sleep safe assessment, Tayyaba, a mother of three, explained to her parent educator that she was unable to purchase a crib for her 2-month-old child, Muhammad, due to financial limitations. Tayyaba's parent educator was able to purchase the family a crib, mattress, sheets, sleep sacks, and pacifiers. The parent educator also informed Tayyaba of the risk of SIDS, the difference between room sharing and bed sharing, how to dress an infant according to the temperature of the home, and more.

One mother who received safe sleep information and a play pen for her infant daughter spoke of the program's impact: "I had limited knowledge on resources in my community, have the barrier of speaking no English, have no family support since everyone is back in Mexico, and since I only have a middle school education, I lacked knowledge on safe sleep, as well. Through All for Kids' Parents as Teachers curriculum, I have learned how to provide safe sleep for my daughter."

For more information on All for Kids and its Safe Sleep Project, visit <www.allforkids.org>.

Putting It Into Practice

- ***Support families in making lifestyle changes.*** Some parents may need to make lifestyle adjustments to support a healthy pregnancy and home environment for an infant. For example, as mentioned earlier in this chapter, smoking during pregnancy is related to increased risk of pregnancy loss, but quitting smoking can be extremely difficult. Support parents in developing and carrying out plans to cut down their smoking, which may include making referrals to healthcare providers or support groups. This is just one example of a lifestyle change that can lead to positive outcomes.
- ***Help families prepare for taking care of an infant.*** Partner with families to prepare safe environments for their infants. Even families who have older children can benefit from reflecting on their previous practices and exploring what, if anything, they would like to do differently this time around. Childproofing and safe sleep are both critical topics for reducing the risk of infant death. Safe sleep, in particular, is often greatly influenced by generational and cultural practices. Initiate conversations by respectfully asking families about their sleep-related beliefs and practices, and where those beliefs and practices originated. Share information about current safe sleep guidelines and the reasons behind them and help families to explore how these guidelines can support safer sleep for their families. For example, current guidelines advise that it is not safe for an adult to sleep while they are holding a baby. Yet, many new parents accidentally fall asleep while holding their babies out of exhaustion, even if they are aware of safe sleep guidelines. Brainstorm with parents ways that they can get more sleep themselves (i.e., leaning on their social support system, taking shifts with a partner) and also avoid accidentally falling asleep while holding their baby (i.e., avoiding sitting alone with baby in a dark room, keeping awake by reading a book or calling a friend).

Your Role as a Community or Social Service Provider

Listening and Learning

As mentioned earlier in this book, even if you are a community or social service provider who does not provide healthcare, it is important that you be informed about issues related to family well-being, health, and access to healthcare. The majority of maternal and infant deaths occur during pregnancy or the postpartum period (versus active labor and delivery), and many of these deaths occur outside of healthcare settings. To this end, you can play a major role in helping your clients: (a) build their understanding of health-related topics; (b) reduce controllable risk factors for themselves and their babies; (c) effectively and confidently advocate for their own physical and mental healthcare needs; and (d) access care in a timely manner.

Advocating

You can also make a difference by translating your experiences with families to systemic advocacy – particularly if you have worked with families who have experienced pregnancy-related deaths or loss. For example, you can draw attention to death rates and unequal access to healthcare in your local community. Your professional and lived experience, coupled with knowledge of basic research and statistics on these issues, can make a compelling case for change.

Amber and Tori's Stories: Imagining Different Endings

The deaths of Amber and Tori were heartbreaking and likely preventable – not because of anything they did wrong, but because of the gaps and inequities in our healthcare and social service systems. Now, imagine that Amber and her fiancé Bruce had a parent educator who could have reinforced their concerns and supported them in finding a more culturally sensitive and trustworthy healthcare provider. Imagine if Tori had a home visitor who could have taken the time to build a trusting relationship with her, provide her with education about what to expect during pregnancy and childbirth, reinforce her connections to her social support system, and connect her to caring medical and mental healthcare providers.

We will never know if the endings to their stories might have been different; however, there are countless others like Amber and Tori for whom community and social service providers could make a life-saving difference.

Take Time to Reflect

Reflecting on the preceding "Putting It Into Practice," what is one area where you believe you are already doing an excellent job? What is one area where you could improve your professional practice or deepen your knowledge and understanding?

Take Action

Now that you have reflected on an area where you could improve your professional practice, create a SMART goal to make it happen. Remember, a SMART goal is described as follows.

- **S**pecific
- **M**easurable
- **A**chievable
- **R**elevant
- Time-Bound

For example, imagine that you would like to collect more handouts and resources on safe sleep that you can share with your pregnant and postpartum clients. A SMART goal might be:

> Safe sleep practices are very important for keeping babies safe (**Relevant**). This month (**Time-Bound**), I will search online for high-quality handouts and resources on safe sleep that I can share with my clients (**Specific, Achievable**). I will print them out and give copies to every pregnant or postpartum client I see this month **(Measurable)**.

Key Takeaways From This Chapter

1. In the United States and similar settings, maternal and infant deaths are most likely to occur during pregnancy and seven or more days after childbirth (versus during active labor and delivery). The vast majority of these deaths are considered preventable.
2. Some groups are more likely to die during and after pregnancy (i.e., people with pre-pregnancy physical or mental health problems, people of color). This is largely due to societal inequalities in healthcare access and quality and other SDOH.
3. Community and social service providers can play an important role in reducing the risk of preventable death during pregnancy, the postpartum period, and the first year of life, even if they do not provide healthcare. The strong relationships that they build with families over time put them in a strong position to provide relevant information to families, to coach self-advocacy skills, and to partner with families to explore ways to keep their children safe.

References

1. McIntyre, B., III (2021). *Amber Rose Isaac*. https://docs.house.gov/meetings/GO/GO00/20210506/112580/HHRG-117-GO00-20210506-SD001.pdf
2. Aponte, C. I. (2021, April). "Every day I wake up fighting for her": A year after the child birth death of Amber Rose Isaac, what's changed? *The City*. www.thecity.nyc/2021/04/20/year-after-childbirth-death-of-amber-rose-isaac-whats-changed/
3. Chappell, B. (2023, June). Tori Bowie, an elite Olympic athlete, died of complications from childbirth. *NPR*. www.npr.org/2023/06/13/1181971448/tori-bowie-an-elite-olympic-athlete-died-of-complications-from-childbirth

4. Fleszar, L. G., Bryant, A. S., Johnson, C. O., Blacker, B. F., Aravkin, A., Baumann, M., Dwyer-Lindgren, L., Kelly, Y. O., Maass, K., Zheng, P., & Roth, G. A. (2023). Trends in state-level maternal mortality by racial and ethnic group in the United States. *JAMA*, *330*(1), 52–61. https://doi.org/10.1001/jama.2023.9043
5. Dattani, S. (2024). *The rise in reported maternal mortality rates in the US is largely due to a change in measurement*. https://ourworldindata.org/rise-us-maternal-mortality-rates-measurement
6. Hoyert, D. L. (2022). *Maternal mortality rates in the United States, 2022*. www.cdc.gov/nchs/data/hestat/maternal-mortality/2022/maternal-mortality-rates-2022.pdf. Accessed December 2024.
7. Trost, S. L., Beauregard, J., Njie, F., et al. (2022). *Pregnancy-related deaths: Data from Maternal Mortality Review Committees in 36 US states, 2017–2019*. Centers for Disease Control and Prevention, US Department of Health and Human Services. www.cdc.gov/maternal-mortality/php/data-research/mmrc-2017-2019.html#cdc_research_or_data_summary_suggested_citation-suggested-citation. Accessed December 2024.
8. Moaddab, A., Dildy, G. A., Brown, H. L., Bateni, Z. H., Belfort, M. A., Sangi-Haghpeykar, H., & Clark, S. L. (2018). Health care disparity and pregnancy-related mortality in the United States, 2005–2014. *Obstetrics & Gynecology*, *131*(4), 707–712. https://doi.org/10.1097/AOG.0000000000002534
9. Ozimek, J. A., & Kilpatrick, S. J. (2018). Maternal mortality in the twenty-first century. *Obstetrics and Gynecology Clinics*, *45*(2), 175–186. https://doi.org/10.1016/j.ogc.2018.01.004
10. Wingate, M. S., Smith, R. A., Petrini, J. R., & Barfield, W. D. (2017). Disparities in gestational age-specific fetal mortality rates in the United States, 2009–2013. *Annals of Epidemiology*, *27*(9), 570–574. https://doi.org/10.1016/j.annepidem.2017.08.014
11. Merkt, P. T., Kramer, M. R., Goodman, D. A., Brantley, M. D., Barrera, C. M., Eckhaus, L., & Petersen, E. E. (2021). Urban-rural differences in pregnancy-related deaths, United States, 2011–2016. *American Journal of Obstetrics and Gynecology*, *225*(2), 183.e1–183.e16. https://doi.org/10.1016/j.ajog.2021.02.028
12. Petersen, E. E., Davis, N. L., Goodman, D., Cox, S., Syverson, C., Seed, K., Shapiro-Mendoza, C., Callaghan, W. M., & Barfield, W. (2019). Racial/ethnic disparities in pregnancy-related deaths – United States, 2007–2016. *Morbidity and Mortality Weekly Report*, *68*(35), 762. https://doi.org/10.15585/mmwr.mm6835a3. Accessed December 2024.
13. Kozhimannil, K. B., Interrante, J. D., Tofte, A. N., & Admon, L. K. (2020). Severe maternal morbidity and mortality among indigenous women in the United States. *Obstetrics and Gynecology*, *135*(2), 294. https://doi.org/10.1097/AOG.0000000000003647
14. Fleszar, L. G., Bryant, A. S., Johnson, C. O., Blacker, B. F., Aravkin, A., Baumann, M., Dwyer-Lindgren, L., Kelly, Y. O., Maass, K., Zheng, P., & Roth, G. A. (2023). Trends in state-level maternal mortality by racial and ethnic group in the United States. *JAMA*, *330*(1), 52–61. https://doi.org/10.1001/jama.2023.9043
15. Gemmill, A., Berger, B. O., Crane, M. A., & Margerison, C. E. (2022). Mortality rates among U.S. women of reproductive age, 1999–2019. *American Journal of Preventive Medicine*, *62*(4), 548–557. https://doi.org/10.1016/j.amepre.2021.10.009
16. Declercq, E., & Zephryin, L. (2020, December). *Maternal mortality in the United States: A primer*. www.commonwealthfund.org/publications/issue-brief-report/2020/dec/maternal-mortality-united-states-primer
17. Obeng, C. S., Jackson, F., Brandenburg, D., & Byrd, K. A. (2023). Black/African American women's woes: Women's perspectives of Black/African American maternal mortality in the USA. *Journal of Racial and Ethnic Health Disparities*. https://doi.org/10.1007/s40615-023-01883-0
18. Chin, K., Wendt, A., Bennett, I. M., & Bhat, A. (2022). Suicide and maternal mortality. *Current Psychiatry Reports*, *24*(4), 239–275. https://doi.org/10.1007/s11920-022-01334-3
19. Combellick, J. L., Esmaeili, A., Johnson, A. M., Haskell, S. G., Phibbs, C. S., Manzo, L., & Miller, L. J. (2024). Perinatal mental health and pregnancy-associated mortality: Opportunities for change. *Archives of Women's Mental Health*, *27*(3), 417–424. https://doi.org/10.1007/s00737-023-01404-2
20. Modest, A. M., Prater, L. C., & Joseph, N. T. (2022). Pregnancy-associated homicide and suicide: An analysis of the National Violent Death Reporting System, 2008–2019. *Obstetrics and Gynecology*, *140*(4), 565–573. https://doi.org/10.1097/AOG.0000000000004932
21. Wallace, M. E. (2022). Trends in pregnancy-associated homicide, United States, 2020. *American Journal of Public Health*, *112*(9), 1333–1336. https://doi.org/10.2105/AJPH.2022.306937

22. Suarez, E. A., Huybrechts, K. F., Straub, L., Hernández-Díaz, S., Creanga, A. A., Connery, H. S., Gray, K. J., Vine, S. M., Jones, H. E., & Bateman, B. T. (2023). Postpartum opioid-related mortality in patients with public insurance. *Obstetrics and Gynecology*, *141*(4), 657–665. https://doi.org/10.1097/AOG.0000000000005115
23. Petersen, E. E., Davis, N. L., Goodman, D., Cox, S., Mayes, N., Johnston, E., Syverson, C., Seed, K., Shapiro-Mendoza, C. K., Callaghan, W. M., & Barfield, W. (2019). Vital signs: Pregnancy-related deaths, United States, 2011–2015, and strategies for prevention, 13 states, 2013–2017. *Morbidity and Mortality Weekly Report*, *68*(18), 423. https://doi.org/10.15585/mmwr.mm6818e1. Accessed December 2024.
24. Burgess, A. P., Dongarwar, D., Spigel, Z., Salihu, H. M., Moaddab, A., Clark, S. L., & Fox, K. (2020). Pregnancy-related mortality in the United States, 2003–2016: Age, race, and place of death. *American Journal of Obstetrics and Gynecology*, *222*(5), 489-e1. https://doi.org/10.1016/j.ajog.2020.02.020
25. Zivin, K., Zhong, C., Rodriguez-Putnam, A., Spring, E., Cai, Q., Miller, A., Johns, L., Kalesnikava, V. A., Courant, A., & Mezuk, B. (2024). Suicide mortality during the perinatal period. *JAMA Network Open*, *7*(6), e2418887. https://doi.org/10.1001/jamanetworkopen.2024.18887
26. Wang, S., Rexrode, K. M., Florio, A. A., Rich-Edwards, J. W., & Chavarro, J. E. (2023). Maternal mortality in the United States: Trends and opportunities for prevention. *Annual Review of Medicine*, *74*, 199–216. https://doi.org/10.1146/annurev-med-042921-123851
27. Wallace, M., Dyer, L., Felker-Kantor, E., Benno, J., Vilda, D., Harville, E., & Theall, K. (2021). Maternity care deserts and pregnancy-associated mortality in Louisiana. *Women's Health Issues*, *31*(2), 122–129. https://doi.org/10.1016/j.whi.2020.09.004
28. U.S. Department of Health and Human Services, Office of Disease Prevention and Health Promotion (n.d.). *Healthy people 2030*. https://health.gov/healthypeople/objectives-and-data/social-determinants-health. Accessed December 2024.
29. Brennan, R. A., & Keohane, C. A. (2016). How communication among members of the health care team affects maternal morbidity and mortality. *Journal of Obstetric, Gynecologic & Neonatal Nursing*, *45*(6), 878–884. https://doi.org/10.1016/j.jogn.2016.03.142
30. Logsdon, M. C., Davis, D. W., Myers, J. A., Masterson, K. M., Rushton, J. A., & Lauf, A. P. (2018). Do new mothers understand the risk factors for maternal mortality? *MCN: The American Journal of Maternal/Child Nursing*, *43*(4), 201–205. https://doi.org/10.1097/NMC.0000000000000434
31. Ganatra, B., & Faundes, A. (2016). Role of birth spacing, family planning services, safe abortion services and post-abortion care in reducing maternal mortality. *Best Practice & Research Clinical Obstetrics & Gynaecology*, *36*, 145–155. https://doi.org/10.1016/j.bpobgyn.2016.07.008
32. Leslie, E. T., & Buntin, M. B. (2018). A systematic approach to translating evidence into practice to reduce infant mortality. *Maternal and Child Health Journal*, *22*(11), 1550–1555. https://doi.org/10.1007/s10995-018-2608-9
33. Addante, A. N., Eisenberg, D. L., Valentine, M. C., Leonard, J., Maddox, K. E. J., & Hoofnagle, M. H. (2021). The association between state-level abortion restrictions and maternal mortality in the United States, 1995–2017. *Contraception*, *104*(5), 496–501. https://doi.org/10.1016/j.contraception.2021.03.018
34. Vilda, D., Wallace, M. E., Daniel, C., Evans, M. G., Stoecker, C., & Theall, K. P. (2021). State abortion policies and maternal death in the United States, 2015–2018. *American Journal of Public Health*, *111*(9), 1696–1704. https://doi.org/10.2105/AJPH.2021.306396
35. Centers for Disease Control and Prevention (n.d.). *About stillbirth*. www.cdc.gov/stillbirth/about/index.html
36. World Health Organization (n.d.). *Why we need to talk about losing a baby*. www.who.int/newsroom/spotlight/why-we-need-to-talk-about-losing-a-baby
37. National Center for Health Statistics (2024). *Infant mortality dashboard*. www.cdc.gov/nchs/nvss/vsrr/infant-mortality-dashboard.htm#:~:text=The%20neonatal%20mortality%20rate%20refers,months%20per%201%2C000%20live%20births. Accessed December 2024.
38. Ely, D. M., & Driscoll, A. K. (2023, November). *Infant mortality in the United States: Provisional data from the 2022 period linked birth/infant death file*. www.cdc.gov/nchs/data/vsrr/vsrr033.pdf. Accessed December 2024.
39. Huang, R., Spence, A. R., & Abenhaim, H. A. (2024). National SIDS trends in the United States from 2000 to 2019: A population-based study on 80 million live births. *Clinical Pediatrics*, *63*(9), 1216–1224. https://doi.org/10.1177/00099228231218162

40. Hwang, S. S., Bourque, S. L., Hannan, K. E., Passarella, M., Radack, J., Formanowski, B., & Lorch, S. A. (2023). Racial and ethnic disparities in sudden unexpected infant death among US infants born preterm. *The Journal of Pediatrics*, *260*, 113498. https://doi.org/10.1016/j.jpeds.2023.113498
41. Atkins, R., Pontes, N. M. H., Patterson, N. A., Hinckson, A., Aromolaran, D., McCray, A., & Pontes, M. C. F. (2024). The effects of race, ethnicity, and maternal education on infant mortality. *Nursing Research*, *73*(1), 37–45. https://doi.org/10.1097/NNR.0000000000000700
42. Owens-Young, J., & Bell, C. N. (2020). Structural racial inequities in socioeconomic status, urban-rural classification, and infant mortality in US counties. *Ethnicity & Disease*, *30*(3), 389. https://doi.org/10.18865/ed.30.3.389
43. Pabayo, R., Cook, D. M., Harling, G., Gunawan, A., Rosenquist, N. A., & Muennig, P. (2019). State-level income inequality and mortality among infants born in the United States 2007–2010: A cohort study. *BMC Public Health*, *19*(1), 1–9. https://doi.org/10.1186/s12889-019-7651-y
44. Janevic, T., Zeitlin, J., Egorova, N. N., Hebert, P., Balbierz, A., Stroustrup, A. M., & Howell, E. A. (2021). Racial and economic neighborhood segregation, site of delivery, and morbidity and mortality in neonates born very preterm. *The Journal of Pediatrics*, *235*, 116–123. https://doi.org/10.1016/j.jpeds.2021.03.049
45. Vilda, D., Hardeman, R., Dyer, L., Theall, K. P., & Wallace, M. (2021). Structural racism, racial inequities and urban-rural differences in infant mortality in the US. *Journal of Epidemiology and Community Health*, *75*(8), 788–793. https://doi.org/10.1136/jech-2020-214260
46. Wallace, M., Crear-Perry, J., Richardson, L., Tarver, M., & Theall, K. (2017). Separate and unequal: Structural racism and infant mortality in the US. *Health & Place*, *45*, 140–144. https://doi.org/10.1016/j.healthplace.2017.03.012
47. Howell, E. A., Janevic, T., Hebert, P. L., Egorova, N. N., Balbierz, A., & Zeitlin, J. (2018). Differences in morbidity and mortality rates in black, white, and Hispanic very preterm infants among New York City hospitals. *JAMA Pediatrics*, *172*(3), 269–277. https://doi.org/10.1001/jamapediatrics.2017.4402
48. Moon, R. Y., & Task Force on Sudden Infant Death Syndrome. (2016). SIDS and other sleep-related infant deaths: Evidence base for 2016 updated recommendations for a safe infant sleeping environment. *Pediatrics*, *138*(5). https://doi.org/10.1542/peds.2016-2940
49. Maged, M., & Rizzolo, D. (2018). Preventing sudden infant death syndrome and other sleep-related infant deaths. *Journal of the American Academy of PAs*, *31*(11), 25–30. https://doi.org/10.1097/01.JAA.0000546475.33947.44
50. Parks, S. E., DeSisto, C. L., Kortsmit, K., Bombard, J. M., & Shapiro-Mendoza, C. K. (2023). Risk factors for suffocation and unexplained causes of infant deaths. *Pediatrics*, *151*(1), e2022057771. https://doi.org/10.1542/peds.2022-057771
51. Salada, K. O., & Badke, C. M. (2022). Missed opportunities: Healthcare encounters prior to sudden unexpected infant death. *Frontiers in Pediatrics*, *10*, 880713. https://doi.org/10.3389/fped.2022.880713
52. Sauber-Schatz, E. K., Sappenfield, W. M., & Shapiro-Mendoza, C. K. (2015). Comprehensive review of sleep-related sudden unexpected infant deaths and their investigations: Florida 2008. *Maternal and Child Health Journal*, *19*(2), 381–390. https://doi.org/10.1007/s10995-014-1520-1
53. Gupta, P. M., Freedman, A. A., Kramer, M. R., Goldenberg, R. L., Willinger, M., Stoll, B. J., Silver, R. M., Dudley, D. J., Parker, C. B., & Hogue, C. J. (2019). Interpregnancy interval and risk of stillbirth: A population-based case control study. *Annals of Epidemiology*, *35*, 35–41. https://doi.org/10.1016/j.annepidem.2019.05.001
54. Ahrens, K. A., Rossen, L. M., & Branum, A. M. (2016). Pregnancy loss history at first parity and selected adverse pregnancy outcomes. *Annals of Epidemiology*, *26*(7), 474–481. https://doi.org/10.1016/j.annepidem.2016.04.011
55. Lamont, K., Scott, N. W., Jones, G. T., & Bhattacharya, S. (2015). Risk of recurrent stillbirth: Systematic review and meta-analysis. *BMJ*, *350*. https://doi.org/10.1136/bmj.h3080
56. Fockler, M. E., Ladhani, N. N. N., Watson, J., & Barrett, J. F. (2017, June). Pregnancy subsequent to stillbirth: Medical and psychosocial aspects of care. In *Seminars in fetal and neonatal medicine* (Vol. 22, No. 3, pp. 186–192). WB Saunders. https://doi.org/10.1016/j.siny.2017.02.004
57. Randolph, A. L., Hruby, B. T., & Sharif, S. (2015). Counseling women who have experienced pregnancy loss: A review of the literature. *Adultspan Journal*, *14*(1), 2–10. https://doi.org/10.1002/j.2161-0029.2015.00032.x

58. Huff, K., Rose, R. S., & Engle, W. A. (2019). Late preterm infants: Morbidities, mortality, and management recommendations. *Pediatric Clinics*, *66*(2), 387–402. https://doi.org/10.1016/j.pcl.2018.12.008
59. Ahrens, K. A., Rossen, L. M., Thoma, M. E., Warner, M., & Simon, A. E. (2017). Birth order and injury-related infant mortality in the US. *American Journal of Preventive Medicine*, *53*(4), 412–420. https://doi.org/10.1016/j.amepre.2017.04.018
60. Thoma, M. E., Rossen, L. M., De Silva, D. A., Warner, M., Simon, A. E., Moskosky, S., & Ahrens, K. A. (2019). Beyond birth outcomes: Interpregnancy interval and injury-related infant mortality. *Paediatric and Perinatal Epidemiology*, *33*(5), 360–370. https://doi.org/10.1111/ppe.12575
61. Bairoliya, N., & Fink, G. (2018). Causes of death and infant mortality rates among full-term births in the United States between 2010 and 2012: An observational study. *PLoS Medicine*, *15*(3), e1002531. https://doi.org/10.1371/journal.pmed.1002531
62. Hauck, F. R., & Blackstone, S. R. (2022). Maternal smoking, alcohol and recreational drug use and the risk of SIDS among a US urban Black population. *Frontiers in Pediatrics*, *10*, 809966. https://doi.org/10.3389/fped.2022.809966
63. Henry, C. J., Higgins, M., Carlson, N., & Song, M. K. (2021). Racial disparities in stillbirth risk factors among non-Hispanic Black women and non-Hispanic white women in the United States. *MCN. The American Journal of Maternal Child Nursing*, *46*(6), 352–359. https://doi.org/10.1097/NMC.0000000000000772
64. Anderson, T. M., Ferres, J. M. L., Ren, S. Y., Moon, R. Y., Goldstein, R. D., Ramirez, J. M., & Mitchell, E. A. (2019). Maternal smoking before and during pregnancy and the risk of sudden unexpected infant death. *Pediatrics*, *143*(4). https://doi.org/10.1542/peds.2018-3325
65. Browne, K., Park, B. Y., Goetzinger, K. R., Caughey, A. B., & Yao, R. (2021). The joint effects of obesity and pregestational diabetes on the risk of stillbirth. *The Journal of Maternal-Fetal & Neonatal Medicine*, *34*(3), 332–338. https://doi.org/10.1080/14767058.2019.1607287
66. Dongarwar, D., Ajewole, V., Spooner, K. K., Tran, V., Adebusuyi, T., Onyenaka, C., Bakare, O., Emeh, C., Baines, K., Boua, D., Mossi, Y., Egbejimi, A., Ibrahim, S., Olaleye, O., & Salihu, H. M. (2024). Racial and ethnic disparities in stillbirth among pregnant women with obesity. *American Journal of Perinatology*, *41*(S 01), e2138–e2144. https://doi.org/10.1055/a-2099-8494
67. Office of Juvenile Justice and Delinquency Prevention (2024). Characteristics of fatality victims of child maltreatment. *OJJDP Statistical Briefing Book*. https://ojjdp.ojp.gov/statistical-briefing-book/victims/faqs/qa02109#:~:text=Infants%20and%20toddlers%20(ages%200,were%20the%20result%20of%20neglect
68. Centers for Disease Control and Prevention (2024, May). *Child abuse and neglect prevention: Risk and protective factors*. www.cdc.gov/child-abuse-neglect/risk-factors/index.html. Accessed December 2024.
69. Wallace, L. A., Rucks, A. C., Ginter, P. M., & Katholi, C. R. (2021). Social factors and public policies associated with state infant mortality rates. *Women & Health*, *61*(4), 337–344. https://doi.org/10.1080/03630242.2021.1889737
70. Bhatt, C. B., & Beck-Sagué, C. M. (2018). Medicaid expansion and infant mortality in the United States. *American Journal of Public Health*, *108*(4), 565–567. https://doi.org/10.2105/AJPH.2017.304218
71. Soneji, S., & Beltrán-Sánchez, H. (2019). Association of special supplemental nutrition program for women, infants, and children with preterm birth and infant mortality. *JAMA Network Open*, *2*(12), e1916722–e1916722. https://doi.org/10.1001/jamanetworkopen.2019.16722
72. Renbarger, K. M., Abebe, S., Place, J. M., Goldsby, E., Hall, G., & Kroot, A. (2023). Perspectives of infant mortality from African American community members. *Women's Health Reports*, *4*(1), 423–430. https://doi.org/10.1089/whr.2023.0017

6 Healthcare During the Preconception Period and Pregnancy

> **Self-Care Moment**
>
> Practicing gratitude is a simple way to enhance your mental and physical well-being. Take a moment to think of three things in your life that you are grateful for, big or small.

The path to healthy pregnancy outcomes begins before conception. Pregnancy planning and healthcare during preconception (before pregnancy), inter-conception (between pregnancies), and pregnancy are all important factors.[1],[2] It is important for community and social service providers to be aware of key issues related to healthcare during these periods, even though they are not usually the ones providing such services. This chapter addresses these topics, including a discussion of relevant research, practice implications for your work, and reflections on your role as a community or social service provider. You will also hear the stories of Caroline, a mother of four weighing her family planning options; Alejandra, an adolescent seeking prenatal care; and several PAT home visiting program affiliates that have woven doula care into their services.

Research Summary

> **Key Terms**
>
> **Family planning**: "The ability of individuals and couples to anticipate and attain their desired number of children, and to plan for the spacing and timing of their births."[3]
>
> **Contraception (also known as birth control)**: Contraception is the act of preventing pregnancy. This can be done by using a device (e.g., an intrauterine device [IUD], contraceptive implant, diaphragm, or condom), taking a medication (e.g., "the pill"), undergoing a procedure (i.e., tubal ligation for people with uteruses), or through a behavior (e.g., abstaining from sexual intercourse altogether or during certain times of one's menstrual cycle with the intention of preventing pregnancy).[4]

DOI: 10.4324/9781003476474-6

Unintended pregnancy: An unintended pregnancy is a pregnancy that is unplanned. This includes situations when the pregnant individual wanted to become pregnant someday but not at this specific time, and situations when the pregnant individual did not want to have any children or any more children.
Preconception care: Medical care provided in preparation for a possible upcoming pregnancy.
Inter-pregnancy interval (IPI): The length of time between when one pregnancy ends and another begins, regardless of pregnancy outcomes.
Inter-pregnancy contraception: Use of contraception between pregnancies to prevent unintended pregnancy.
Miscarriage: Natural loss of a pregnancy before the 20th week of gestation.

Preconception Healthcare, Family Planning, and Contraception

Preconception Healthcare

It is important that all people of childbearing age receive regular preventive medical care and guidance about unique aspects of their health or lifestyle that could affect any future pregnancies.[5] Preconception healthcare and education occurs before an individual (or their partner) becomes pregnant – with a focus on optimizing health, addressing risk factors, and providing education about how to increase the chances of a healthy pregnancy. This includes education about sexual health, coaching around components of a healthy lifestyle (i.e., a balanced diet, smoking cessation), and treatment for chronic conditions such as high blood pressure, depression, or substance misuse.[6,7] Depending on the individual's unique health needs and how far in advance they wish to plan pregnancy, these forms of healthcare and education can begin long before a pregnancy is conceived.

The American College of Obstetricians and Gynecologists also recommends that anyone who is planning to get pregnant soon participate in a preconception check-up – regardless of past pregnancy history.[8] Ideally, a preconception check-up with a healthcare provider occurs within a few months of beginning to try to get pregnant. This typically includes a physical exam; review of previous health, pregnancy, and vaccination histories; discussion about any lifestyle changes that need to be made in preparation for pregnancy (i.e., discontinuing certain medications or substances, or starting to take new medications or supplements, such as prenatal vitamins); guidance around conception and what to expect in the early stages of pregnancy; and education about potential health warning signs to look out for in early pregnancy.[9]

Despite supporting positive maternal and child health outcomes, access to high-quality preconception healthcare and education is often limited and varies based on factors such as a patient's age, health literacy, marital status, income, immigration status, and other factors.[10] Research on preconception care suggests that healthcare providers do not consistently discuss pre-pregnancy health issues or pregnancy planning with their patients before they conceive.[11,12] Additionally, traditional preconception healthcare routines often exclude men, despite a growing body of research suggesting that male preconception health affects both infant and maternal outcomes.[13,14,15]

Putting It Into Practice

- ***Reinforce the importance of regular preventive healthcare.*** Discuss the importance of regular preventive care and its relationship to preconception health with all clients of reproductive age. Within your role, you likely have more time than healthcare providers to explore the reasons why someone may not be engaging in regular healthcare. Sometimes, people do not get regular preventive or preconception healthcare not because they are reluctant, but because they do not have health insurance or a medical home. When you are knowledgeable about options in your local community, you can support your clients in accessing more regular healthcare services.
- ***Help to address roadblocks to timely, attentive healthcare services.*** Unfortunately, it is common for people to feel unheard by their healthcare providers, and to experience other roadblocks to timely, attentive care. These experiences are particularly common for people of color, people with lower socioeconomic resources, and other groups. You can validate the reality of these experiences and work with families as they advocate for and make decisions related to their own healthcare. You can help bridge communication gaps between healthcare providers and the people you work with by supporting them in identifying and articulating their questions, concerns, and wishes. This could include roleplaying and/or practicing conversations in advance of appointments with healthcare providers.

Caroline's Story ♥

Caroline and her husband Danny always wanted a big family – they just didn't expect to have one so quickly. By the time they were both 26 years old, they had four children – ages 5 years, 4 years, 2 years, and 6 months. They loved each of their children, but Caroline's last pregnancy was physically and mentally challenging, and their finances were becoming strained. Caroline was nervous about the possibility of getting pregnant again, but she was also nervous about birth control. She did not like the idea of taking medication and had heard about possible side effects. She considered setting up an appointment with her gynecologist but hesitated when she remembered the judgmental looks that she received the last time she came into the clinic with all four children.

Take Time to Reflect

As a community or social service professional, how comfortable do you feel asking your clients about their family planning goals and timelines? How do your personal, cultural, religious, or other beliefs/values play a role?

Family Planning Conversations

In the United States, a little less than half of pregnancies are unintended.[16] Family planning can help individuals and couples time pregnancy when they are ready for it emotionally, physically, financially, and otherwise. Planned pregnancies tend to be associated with lower stress, fewer risk factors, and better maternal and infant outcomes compared to unplanned pregnancies. Contraceptive use before conception is also associated with lower risk of severe health complications for those with pre-existing chronic health conditions.[17]

While many unintended pregnancies ultimately result in healthy babies and parents, there are some additional risks associated with them. Pregnancies that are unintended have been linked to delayed prenatal care, higher rates of intimate partner violence during pregnancy, premature birth, and low birthweight.[18,19] Research has also found that unintended pregnancy is associated with significantly increased risk of depression during pregnancy and the postpartum period.[20] (For additional information about supporting the mental health of parents/caregivers who may be experiencing an unplanned pregnancy, refer to Chapter 3.)

Family planning is important not only for first pregnancies, but also for planning the timing between pregnancies for parents who want more than one child, and for preventing subsequent pregnancies for those who do not want to become pregnant again. Despite common misconceptions, it is possible to become pregnant within three weeks after giving birth – even when breastfeeding.[21] Therefore, it is also important that family planning conversations occur during pregnancy or early in the postpartum period to ensure healthy inter-pregnancy intervals (or, spacing between pregnancies). Adequate spacing between pregnancies allows for physical and mental recovery before becoming pregnant again, which can reduce the risk of complications in subsequent pregnancies.[22,23]

In general, the American College of Obstetricians and Gynecologists recommends that there be no less than 18 months and no more than five years between the end of one pregnancy and the start of another.[22] Other groups like the World Health Organization (WHO) offer similar guidelines. When there is less time between pregnancies, there is a higher risk for maternal and infant health complications, such as preterm birth, premature rupture of membranes, low birthweight and small size for gestational age, infant birth injuries, severe maternal complications, and infant and maternal death.[24,25,26,27] Meanwhile, longer-than-recommended spacing between pregnancies has been linked to an increased risk of complications such as induction of labor, unplanned C-section, severe maternal complications, maternal intensive care unit admissions, and preterm delivery.[27,28]

Despite the general guidance previously listed, there are variations in recommended spacing between pregnancies based on birth outcomes and other factors. Research suggests that becoming pregnant within six months of live childbirth is associated with increased risk of negative health outcomes. However, for those who have experienced a miscarriage (a natural loss of a pregnancy before the 20th week of gestation), getting pregnant within six months appears to be related to reduced risk of subsequent miscarriage and preterm delivery.[29,30] Pregnancy spacing guidelines also differ for individuals who have experienced ectopic pregnancies, stillbirth, C-section, and other conditions. In addition, individuals who are older or who use assisted reproductive technology (i.e., intrauterine insemination [IUI], in-vitro fertilization [IVF], etc.) to get pregnant may need to carefully evaluate the potential risks and benefits of significantly delaying attempts to get pregnant. Because of this, it is essential that parents have a conversation with their healthcare provider about the ideal pregnancy spacing for their unique situation.

In general, there are significant gaps between best practices for contraception use during the postpartum period and what parents know. Continuity of care (i.e., receiving care from the same provider or at the same clinic) from pregnancy through the postpartum period can reduce these gaps and result in more timely use of contraception after giving birth.[31] Age, race, ethnicity, whether the pregnancy was carried to full-term, number of babies, insurance type, and other factors have all been identified as influences on access to postpartum contraceptive counseling.[32] Overall, many people do not receive high-quality counseling about their postpartum contraception options, and are thus more likely to choose no contraception, or less effective or reliable methods (i.e., the withdrawal/"pullout" method, the rhythm method) and to experience unintended pregnancy.[33,34,35] In addition, access to effective, affordable contraception can be a significant challenge. Even if families know about effective contraceptive options, they may not be able to afford or access them.

Studies have also suggested that, for individuals in committed relationships, including both partners in family planning conversations helps to reduce the likelihood of rapid, repeat pregnancy (i.e., conception within 24 months of birth). When possible, healthcare, community, and social service providers should include both partners in family planning discussions to support open communication, dispel myths, and promote each partners' knowledge to make informed decisions related to family planning and contraceptive use.[36]

While family planning is ideally a conversation between partners, there are times when it is driven more by one parent than others. Research has demonstrated that in heterosexual relationships, fathers' intentions have a strong role in reproductive decisions – for example, one study found that the odds of rapid repeat pregnancy was highest when fathers intended pregnancy, even when mothers did not.[36] The authors of this study suggested that women in relationships characterized by male dominance, and those in abusive or controlling relationships, may be at particular risk for having their family planning wishes overturned – pointing to the importance of culturally sensitive interventions and intimate partner violence screenings.

It is important to recognize that beliefs and values related to family planning and contraception vary based on culture, religion, and other factors – including among those reading this book. Some people and groups believe that all methods of contraception are acceptable from moral and health perspectives, others believe that only some methods of contraception are acceptable, and still others believe that all contraceptive methods are unacceptable. Healthcare, community, and social service providers must strike a delicate balance between respecting and working within their clients' values and beliefs, while also providing them with up-to-date information about the role that family planning can play in promoting healthy outcomes.

Putting It Into Practice

- ***Offer a safe, non-judgmental space for people to explore family planning.*** Community and social service providers can provide a safe space for clients to understand the basics of family planning and contraception options, and to explore their preferences. When possible, these conversations can be very helpful to have before people meet with their healthcare provider, so that they can prepare for the appointment and be ready to receive more detailed medical information and guidance. If the person does not have a consistent healthcare provider, you can help identify and facilitate a connection.

- ***Pay close attention to emotional and physical safety.*** If a pregnant or postpartum client has a supportive partner, you can engage them in these conversations to further support family planning activities and avoid unintended pregnancies. However, you should remain attentive to any information you have received and your professional observations about the emotional and physical safety of including a partner in these conversations.
- ***Make the connection to mental health.*** People who have previously experienced trauma or who are currently experiencing mental health challenges (such as depression and anxiety) may be more likely to engage in high-risk sexual behaviors, making them more vulnerable to unintended pregnancy. This highlights the importance of mental health screening and history-taking with all clients as a means of supporting family planning. It can be beneficial to have a supportive conversation and provide basic education about mental health before conducting a screening. In addition, when a screening suggests that someone may be struggling with their mental health, it is best practice to offer referrals and/or resources (i.e., crisis hotline numbers). This may require some creativity in communities where resources are limited – for example, connecting people with telehealth options or primary care providers, or offering a mental health intervention that is designed to be implemented in community settings by providers who are not mental health professionals.

Take Time to Reflect

As a community or social service professional, how can you ensure that you approach conversations about family planning in a non-judgmental, culturally humble way? What types of resources or support would help to build your skill and comfort?

Prenatal Healthcare

Once a pregnancy is conceived, early and regular prenatal healthcare is essential to promoting healthy outcomes.[37] For pregnancies with limited risk, the American Academy of Pediatrics and the American College of Obstetricians and Gynecologists recommend that prenatal visits occur monthly between conception and 28 weeks gestation, every other week between 28 and 36 weeks gestation, and at least weekly from 36 weeks until delivery.[38]

Unfortunately, research indicates that many prenatal healthcare experiences do not align with recommended guidelines. In the United States, it has been estimated that about one-quarter of pregnant individuals do not access prenatal healthcare until after the first trimester.[39] Delays in accessing prenatal care can be related to many factors, such as unintended pregnancy, lack of nearby healthcare facilities, and/or difficulties finding the time, transportation, or other resources needed to attend healthcare appointments, to name a few.[40]

Delayed prenatal healthcare is particularly concerning for those with unintended pregnancies and/or who did not receive preconception care. These individuals may be particularly likely to have health or lifestyle factors that need to be addressed as soon as possible (i.e., preconception diabetes, hypertension, ongoing substance use, medication usage, lack of prenatal vitamins).[41] Given increasing regional restrictions, delays in early prenatal healthcare may also limit the healthcare options available to individuals who cannot continue their pregnancy for any number of reasons.

Overall, inadequate prenatal healthcare has been linked to increased risk of various negative health outcomes during pregnancy, the postpartum period, and the first year of life – for example, insufficient gestational weight gain, early labor, premature rupture of membranes, low infant birthweight, and neonatal intensive care admission.[42,43,44,45] On the other hand, a systematic review of multiple studies found that prenatal healthcare was an important factor in reducing the occurrence of pregnancy-related health complications like hypertension or high blood pressure.[46] Another study of pregnant women with pre-gestational diabetes found that those who received treatment for diabetes throughout pregnancy were less likely to experience negative outcomes, such as death of the baby before birth.[47]

Prenatal Vaccination

Vaccinations are a vital aspect of prenatal care that help to protect pregnant individuals and their babies from illness.[48,49,50,51,52] As of 2022, the American College of Obstetricians and Gynecologists recommended that prenatal healthcare routinely include vaccination for influenza (the flu), tetanus toxoid/reduced diptheria toxoid/acellular pertussis (Tdap), and COVID-19; and that certain groups receive pneumococcal, meningococcal, and/or Hepatitis A and B vaccines.[52] Prenatal RSV vaccination or, alternatively, giving babies antibodies upon birth, is also recommended.[52]

Extensive research indicates that these recommended vaccinations are safe during pregnancy and have no adverse effects on birth outcomes. Research on the influenza vaccine has demonstrated no association between prenatal vaccination and adverse birth outcomes; and in fact, prenatal influenza vaccination has been linked to lower likelihood of health complications during pregnancy such as fever, preeclampsia, placental abruption, stillbirth, and NICU admission.[53,54] Another study indicated that prenatal influenza vaccination provides antibody protection not only to the individual who receives the vaccine, but also to their infant through three months of age.[55] Despite these promising findings, vaccination rates remain low during pregnancy. For example, nationally representative data from the United States indicated that less than half – and perhaps as few as one-third – of pregnant patients during 2012–2016 received influenza vaccinations.[56,57]

Many factors affect prenatal vaccination rates, including personal beliefs.[58,59,60] One study indicated that nearly half of pregnant women were declining routine prenatal vaccines, and that the most common reasons were believing that vaccines were ineffective or unimportant, and concerns about possible adverse effects on their baby.[61] Other research has found that health beliefs have a bigger effect on vaccination decisions during pregnancy than demographics and other factors.[62,63]

Healthcare, community, and social service providers all play important roles in educating families about the importance of prenatal vaccinations and addressing any concerns or questions they might have. Several studies have identified unique interventions in this domain, such as Text4Baby – a free national text-messaging system that sends encouraging messages around receiving prenatal influenza vaccinations – and web-based vaccination information, such as educational websites and social media.[64,65,66]

Take Action

If you work with pregnant clients, it is important that you stay up to date with routine vaccinations, such as ones for influenza and RSV, to help keep your clients and yourself safe. Schedule an appointment with your local healthcare provider or pharmacy today.

Dental Care

Another important aspect of prenatal healthcare is dental care. Routine dental care is safe to continue during pregnancy, and is important for reducing lifelong risk of cardiovascular disease, diabetes, and other diseases.[67] Furthermore, although normal, changes to the gums and teeth during pregnancy increase the risk of developing conditions such as pregnancy gingivitis, tooth erosion, dental caries, and periodontitis.[67] Prompt identification and treatment of these conditions is important for health and comfort, and may also reduce the risk of transmitting caries-producing oral bacteria to infants after birth.

Despite these findings, many people are unaware of the importance of dental care during pregnancy. Many others are unable to access dental care due to financial strain, lack of dental insurance, or other factors.[67] One study found that only 47% of women visited a dentist in the 12 months before getting pregnant, and that this rate was lower for individuals in their 20s, those with lower levels of education, and those identifying with certain racial and ethnic groups.[68] General anxiety around dental care has also been linked to lower likelihood of visiting the dentist during pregnancy.[69]

Disparities in Healthcare Access and Patient–Provider Relationships

Despite the importance of quality prenatal healthcare, many are not able to access timely and sufficient care during pregnancy. Access to care varies widely based on factors like income, race and ethnicity, geographic location, age, education level, immigration status, disability status, and psychosocial stressors.[70,71] One study that examined nine years of birth records from the city and county of St. Louis, Missouri indicated that Black individuals, adolescents, those with fewer than 13 years of education, and public insurance recipients were less likely to receive adequate prenatal care than other groups.[44] Similarly, a study of live births across several years in California found that those who were younger, those with fewer than 12 years of education, public insurance recipients, and those who struggled with drug or alcohol use were more likely to enter prenatal care later in their pregnancies.[72] Other work has reported that pregnant refugees are more likely to start prenatal care later than recommended.[73]

Barriers to appropriate and timely prenatal care also disproportionally affect pregnant individuals living in remote and low-resource areas.[74,75,76] One study across the United

States found that between 2002 and 2013, the geographic distribution of hospital obstetric units and advanced neonatal care facilities was uneven. Specifically, pregnant individuals who lived in rural areas or in counties with lower incomes and levels of educational attainment had to travel further to access prenatal care.[77] Another study found that between 2004 and 2014, 9% of rural counties in the United States experienced reductions in hospital obstetric services, and another 45% had no local obstetric services at all.[78] The same study found that non-Hispanic Black women of childbearing age were more likely to live in areas where there were fewer obstetricians and physicians nearby, and that those with lower incomes and/or public insurance were more likely to have difficulty accessing hospital-based obstetric services.[78]

Those with disabilities also face significant barriers to appropriate and timely prenatal care. In a study of Massachusetts childbirths from 1998–2010, women with intellectual and developmental disabilities were less likely to receive prenatal care during their first trimester than those without disabilities.[79] Another study conducted surveys of women with physical disabilities.[80] Despite more than half of respondents identifying that they sought out a prenatal healthcare provider who they believed would be sensitive to their disability, 40% of the group reported that their providers ultimately exhibited little to no specialized knowledge about how their specific physical disability might affect their pregnancy – underscoring the need for greater provider training, education, and sensitivity.

Putting It Into Practice

- ***Facilitate access to preventive and prenatal healthcare.*** Community and social service providers can play a valuable role in facilitating access to high-quality, culturally responsive healthcare providers. In addition to being familiar with healthcare options in the community and facilitating connections, you might also assist with supports such as access to transportation and childcare to make attending healthcare appointments possible.
- ***Help pregnant and postpartum clients to process information that they receive during healthcare appointments.*** During pregnancy and the postpartum period, patients and their families often receive a lot of information in a short period of time during healthcare appointments. You can help them process and reinforce this information in a familiar, unhurried setting. They may also feel more comfortable voicing questions and concerns within the safe space and trusting relationship they have with you. You can also help them to prepare for upcoming healthcare appointments by sharing information about what to expect and practicing sharing questions and concerns with a healthcare provider.
- ***Support clients with disabilities in accessing preventive and prenatal care.*** You can support access to care by identifying healthcare professionals who are well-versed in disabilities, or professionals that can accompany people with disabilities to healthcare appointments and offer support. You can also support pregnant clients with disabilities in understanding more about pregnancy and what to expect during prenatal care appointments. If possible, you can offer educational resources that are digestible for people with different types of disabilities (i.e., limited vision, intellectual disabilities).

Screening Pregnant Individuals in the Emergency Department

Participating in routine prenatal care with an established healthcare provider is ideal; however, the emergency department is a critical resource for many during pregnancy, especially those from marginalized backgrounds or those who live in rural areas with limited obstetric care. Studies have found that those who utilize the emergency department for any number of health issues (related to pregnancy or not) tend to have higher levels of psychosocial and health risk factors such as domestic violence, substance misuse, and smoking; chronic health conditions such as asthma, diabetes, hypertension, and obesity; and severe illnesses that are not being adequately addressed at the outpatient level.[81,82,83] Those who frequently utilize unscheduled emergency department care have also reported lower levels of self-efficacy and social support.[83] Screening pregnant patients in the emergency department may be a promising strategy for identifying high-risk individuals with inadequate access to regular prenatal care, and for connecting those individuals to resources and referrals for regular care.

Take Time to Reflect

Think about what you know about prenatal care in your community. What are some strengths of the systems? What do you think may be barriers to accessing quality care? How does (or could) your organization play a role in addressing these challenges?

Patient–Provider Relationships

Alejandra's Story ♥

Alejandra, a 16-year-old Mexican American girl from Texas, was surprised and afraid when she learned that she was pregnant. She did not tell anyone, including her parents, until she was five months along and could not hide her belly anymore. At that point, her mother Luciana brought her to a local healthcare clinic for a prenatal check-up. When the doctor entered the room, she looked at Alejandra's belly with a furrowed brow. "This is your first check-up?" the doctor asked sternly. "Why did you wait so long to come in? Do you understand how risky that was for your baby?"

Alejandra's cheeks flushed. "I . . . I . . . " she stammered, looking to her mother for help. Luciana jumped in and began asking the doctor questions in Spanish.

"Sorry, I don't speak Spanish," the doctor interrupted. "I'm not sure if our interpreter is in today, but I can go check."

Collaborative, trusting patient–provider relationships and effective communication are critically important before, during, and after pregnancy. This is particularly impactful when working with patients who have had negative experiences with the healthcare system in the past, or who have heard stories of others who have.[84,85] To support patient–provider relationships, the American College of Obstetricians and Gynecologists has published evidence-based guidelines that emphasize patient-centered care, developing patient advocacy skills, and sensitivity.[86] Unfortunately, research shows that Black women and other groups of pregnant patients (i.e., those from lower-income backgrounds, those struggling with substance use) continue to experience high levels of discrimination and microaggressions during prenatal care.[87,88,89,90,91,92,93] A large review study found that patients of color commonly reported that their prenatal care providers were discriminatory toward them and/or did not adequately address their questions and information needs.[94]

When patients are involved in a shared decision-making process, it directly affects the likelihood that they will follow recommendations of their healthcare provider. Factors such as a parent's trust in the provider, feelings of self-efficacy, perceived discrimination, perceived compassion and cultural competency of the healthcare provider, and more also indirectly influence whether or not they will follow recommendations.[95,96,97]

Take Time to Reflect

Think about the variety of racial and ethnic backgrounds in your community, including any Indigenous populations. What do you know about cultural beliefs and practices related to pregnancy and prenatal care that differ from yours? How can you learn more in a sensitive and respectful way, so that you can better communicate with all of your pregnant and postpartum clients?

Alternative and Supplementary Care

In recent decades in the United States and similar settings, prenatal healthcare has traditionally occurred in person in healthcare clinics. However, alternative and supplementary care models that go beyond the standard office visit schedule have also been shown to be beneficial for many patients. In fact, studies have found that some of these care models can result in equivalent or even better health outcomes for pregnant patients and their babies, especially those from marginalized backgrounds.[98] In what follows, we briefly discuss four models: (a) group prenatal care; (b) midwifery; (c) telehealth; and (d) doula care.

Group Prenatal Care

Due to heavy caseloads, insurance regulations, and other factors, individual healthcare providers are often forced to have brief appointments with patients. This can have negative effects on patient-centered care and relationship-building between the provider and the family. Group prenatal care is an alternative to traditional care that combines clinical services, education, and peer support. One of the most successful models in the United States is Centering Pregnancy, which brings together small groups of individuals with similar due dates to participate in group appointments with a healthcare provider, lasting between 90 minutes and two hours. These appointments are scheduled at the same intervals as traditional prenatal visits and include brief health assessments with the healthcare provider, as well as group discussions and interactive activities. Research has found that this group prenatal care model is associated with improvements in participants' psychological well-being; decreased risk of preterm birth, low birthweight, and NICU admissions, and becoming pregnant again soon after giving birth; and higher rates of well-child visit attendance after baby is born.[99,100,101] Similarly, evidence has been found across various group prenatal care models that participants feel more satisfied with their care experience and more educated and prepared for birth.[102,103] Research has also found that pregnant adolescents, Black individuals, low-income individuals, and individuals struggling with tobacco or drug use may particularly benefit from group prenatal care.[104]

Midwifery

During pregnancy, many choose to work with midwives for some or all their prenatal care. Certified midwives can support with most aspects of prenatal care, including routine appointments, ultrasounds, and childbirth. In some cultures, midwives who are not professionally certified but who have significant childbirth and cultural knowledge are also commonly relied on. This practice has been found to be safe and effective for many low-risk patients.[105,106] Midwives may be a part of a standard obstetrician/gynecologist healthcare practice or may operate independently. Midwife-led care has also been linked to lower rates of preterm birth.[107] It is important to note that there is some evidence that Black clients may be more likely to leave midwife care mid-pregnancy than individuals from other racial and ethnic backgrounds, which raises questions about the quality and cultural sensitivity of the midwifery services they receive.[108]

Telehealth

Telehealth appointments have become increasingly common since the start of the COVID-19 pandemic in 2020, and prenatal care appointments are no exception.[109] Clinicians and researchers have noted that while telehealth cannot replace all in-person care (for example, appointments at key timepoints in pregnancy that require physical examinations, ultrasounds, bloodwork, gestational diabetes screenings, or vaccinations), it can be a convenient option for appointments that primarily involve patient counseling and education.[110,111,112,113] Insurance coverage of telehealth visits also varies and may be in further flux depending on future legislation. Of course, patient risk status, access to and comfort with technology, local laws, and other factors must also be considered.[110] Research during the COVID-19 pandemic found that the most common reasons that patients did not pursue telehealth visits during pregnancy were preferring in-person appointments, lack of available telehealth appointments, technology barriers, and lack of private space.[114]

Doulas

In response to the growing rate of maternal complications and death in the United States, programs nationwide have recognized the critical impact of integrating doula services into home visiting. Doulas – trained professionals who provide continuous physical, emotional, and informational support during pregnancy, childbirth, and the postpartum period – are now commonly included in perinatal care models, and many programs have seen positive health outcomes as a result. Doulas help to bridge gaps in care by offering personalized support, advocating for patients' needs, and monitoring for potential health risks.

Putting It Into Practice

- ***Increase awareness of the range of healthcare options.*** As a community or social service provider, you likely work across your community and interact with a wide variety of resources and services. Thus, you are well-positioned to share information regarding different types of prenatal services and supports with your clients, such as those described previously. Further, you can help connect pregnant and postpartum families with reputable alternative or supplemental care options in which they are interested.

- ***Facilitate group support.*** As a community or social service provider, you can offer avenues for pregnant and postpartum families to connect with others who are at similar points in their journeys. Groups might be professionally led, led by the participants, or a combination of both. Together, participants can offer each other wisdom and support as they navigate their shared experiences.

Parents as Teachers/Healthy Start Coalition of Pinellas' Wellness Team Δ

In Florida, the Healthy Start Coalition of Pinellas has created a comprehensive "wellness team" approach to support prenatal families by bringing together a range of professionals who address both physical and emotional needs. This team is composed of nurses, mental health counselors, a nutritionist, and a team of certified doulas, each offering specialized support to ensure families receive well-rounded prenatal care.

Key to this model is the inclusion of doulas trained through the G.R.O.W. Doula Program, who bring expertise and advocacy for expecting parents. To further enhance their skills, these doulas participate in a mingling and mentoring program, which connects them with experienced doulas. This mentoring aspect provides them with real-world insights and practical advice, enhancing their ability to support expectant families effectively.

The program has also integrated the following additional prenatal support measures aimed at reducing health risks and increasing parents' preparedness for childbirth and infant care.

Blood Pressure Cuffs: Recognizing the risks posed by hypertension and other comorbidities during pregnancy, the program offers blood pressure cuffs to high-risk clients. Instructing pregnant individuals as to how to use this simple but essential tool allows them to monitor their blood pressure at home, potentially catching early signs of complications like preeclampsia.

Infant CPR Dolls: Expectant families receive infant CPR education and dolls to practice life-saving skills before their baby arrives. This training helps new parents feel more prepared and confident in handling emergencies, which is crucial for families who may not have easy access to immediate medical assistance.

This wellness team approach combines the expertise of healthcare and wellness professionals to ensure comprehensive prenatal support. By addressing various dimensions of health – from mental well-being and nutrition to childbirth education and emergency preparedness – the PAT+/Healthy Start Coalition of Pinellas model is helping families feel supported, informed, and ready for the journey into parenthood.

For more information on PAT+/Healthy Start Coalition of Pinellas and its wellness team approach, visit <healthystartpinellas.org/pat/>.

The Show Me Strong Families Doula Program Δ

One innovative example of how doula work is being integrated into community services is the Show Me Strong Families (SMSF) program, an affiliate of the PATNC in St. Louis, Missouri. Here, five parent educators – four Black, or African American, and one Spanish-speaking Latina – have undergone additional training to become certified as full-spectrum doulas. These doulas demographically reflect the families they serve. The doula training enables them to support families throughout the entire perinatal period, which includes pregnancy, birth, and postpartum. Since beginning services in 2020, SMSF has provided doula support in more than 160 births.

The full-spectrum doulas in this program expand on roles beyond traditional home visiting by focusing on the unique needs and experiences of each birthing person and family. In addition to their regular caseload, they provide specialized visits including the following services.

Monitoring for Maternal Health Risks: These doulas are trained to identify and respond to signs of complications, like high blood pressure or excessive swelling, that may indicate risks such as preeclampsia or postpartum hemorrhage. Early identification of these "red flags" enables quicker intervention, which is crucial in preventing severe health outcomes.

Advocating for Birthing Preferences and Plans: People often feel more confident and empowered when they are supported by someone who understands their goals and can advocate on their behalf during medical visits. SMSF doulas play a key role in supporting birthing plans, ensuring that preferences around delivery methods, pain management, and postpartum care are effectively communicated to medical providers.

Providing Emotional and Educational Support: The doulas serve as a steady source of reassurance and information, helping to ease anxiety and build confidence for new parents. They offer guidance on topics such as breastfeeding, postpartum recovery, and newborn care, helping families feel more prepared and connected.

By combining the educational and supportive elements of home visiting with the personalized, advocacy-driven approach of doula care, SMSF exemplifies a holistic model for perinatal support. This approach not only strengthens maternal and infant health outcomes but also fosters a deeper sense of trust and understanding between families and their support networks. Through models like these, programs nationwide are reshaping perinatal care to create safer, more responsive experiences for families.

Chicanos Por La Causa (CPLC) Parenting Arizona's Doula Program Δ

In response to the lack of accessible maternity and doula services in Arizona's most rural areas, the CPLC Parenting Arizona program has stepped in to provide critical perinatal support to families in these maternity care deserts. Recognizing that distance and scarcity of healthcare providers can leave many expectant parents without essential resources, the program has trained 11 parent educators as doulas to support families throughout pregnancy, birth, and the postpartum period.

This training marks a significant shift in the type of care that Parenting Arizona can offer to its families. These newly trained doulas not only provide guidance through the birth process but have also received specialized training on lactation and breastfeeding support. Within the first six months of the program, these doulas assisted 14 families, offering guidance on feeding techniques and helping mothers overcome breastfeeding challenges – support that is often unavailable in isolated regions.

According to the program manager, doula work involves a deep level of personal connection and trust, as well as a substantial time commitment from the trainees. In a field where healthcare and personal support are often fragmented or hard to access, these doulas have become trusted allies for families, providing continuity and a reliable presence.

This amplified level of support has also had a profound effect on the parent educators themselves. The supervisor notes that through doula training, the educators have become more comfortable and confident in their roles. They enter each home visit with a stronger understanding of perinatal needs, enabling them to offer comprehensive support that extends through pregnancy, labor, delivery, and the early days of parenthood.

Through the addition of doula services, the CPLC Parenting Arizona program has transformed home visiting in rural Arizona, making quality perinatal care accessible in some of the state's most underserved regions. This program is an inspiring example of how training, commitment, and local support can help reduce barriers to maternal and infant health, even in areas where medical resources are scarce.

For more information on CPLC Parenting Arizona and its integration of doula services, visit <https://cplc.org/hhs/parenting.php>.

Your Role as a Community or Social Service Provider

Listening and Learning

The data and information in this chapter show both the importance of and challenges to intentional pregnancy planning and quality preconception and prenatal healthcare. Understanding the data and statistics specific to your community will help you serve as an effective bridge and connector between those you work with and needed community resources and services. Consider: what do you already know about the quality, accessibility and cultural responsiveness of preventive and prenatal healthcare services in your community? What processes do you have for staying up to date with this information, including identifying contacts with whom to make a warm hand-off?

In addition to researching local data and statistics, you can learn a lot from listening to personal stories of the families you work with, as well as other families in your community. How do families' experiences with preventive and prenatal healthcare vary? What are common strengths and challenges among them? Consider: how can you apply what you learn to inform the services you provide?

Advocating

As discussed throughout this book, your role as a community or social service provider operates on two levels: (a) your individual work with families; and (b) your work with systems in your community, including healthcare. The lessons outlined in this chapter pertain to both levels of work and point to the need for broad advocacy for accessible, culturally responsive, high quality healthcare services. Within your organization, you can contribute to the development and maintenance of information about healthcare services in your community that meet these criteria. Whenever possible, it is beneficial for organizations to establish written agreements that facilitate families' timely access to these healthcare services. You can also advocate outside of your organization in the community at large, by lifting up policies, programs, and initiatives that increase the availability and accessibility of quality healthcare regardless of one's ability, geographical location or socioeconomic status.

Take Time to Reflect

Reflecting on the practice implications throughout this chapter and your role as a community or social service provider, what is one area where you believe you are already doing an excellent job? What is one area where you could improve your professional practice or deepen your knowledge and understanding?

Take Action

Now that you have reflected on an area where you could improve your professional practice, create a SMART goal to make it happen. Remember, a SMART goal is described as follows.

- **S**pecific
- **M**easurable
- **A**chievable
- **R**elevant
- **T**ime-Bound

For example, imagine that you would like to become more comfortable and confident in discussing family planning with your clients. A SMART goal might be:

> I know that family planning is an important topic for my clients and their families, though I'm not always sure how to bring it up during our visits (**Relevant**). I will ask my supervisor if we can add this topic to the agenda for our staff meeting later this month, and maybe even do some role-play conversations together (**Time-Bound, Specific, Achievable, Measurable**).

Key Takeaways From This Chapter

1. High-quality, culturally sensitive care during the preconception period and pregnancy is important for maternal and infant health and well-being; however, many groups struggle to access timely and sufficient care due to systematic barriers.
2. People of color, low-income people, and other groups often experience discrimination and substandard prenatal care. Community and social service providers can play an important role in helping these clients to navigate their relationships with healthcare providers and referring them to other healthcare providers when needed.
3. Group prenatal care, midwifery, telehealth, and doulas are all promising alternative and/or supplementary care models.

References

1. Ganatra, B., & Faundes, A. (2016). Role of birth spacing, family planning services, safe abortion services and post-abortion care in reducing maternal mortality. *Best Practice & Research Clinical Obstetrics & Gynaecology*, *36*, 145–155. https://doi.org/10.1016/j.bpobgyn.2016.07.008
2. Leslie, E. T., & Buntin, M. B. (2018). A systematic approach to translating evidence into practice to reduce infant mortality. *Maternal and Child Health Journal*, *22*(11), 1550–1555. https://doi.org/10.1007/s10995-018-2608-9
3. World Health Organization (n.d.). *Contraception*. www.who.int/health-topics/contraception#tab=tab_1
4. Bansode, O. M., Sarao, M. S., & Cooper, D. B. (2023). *Contraception*. StatPearls Publishing. www.ncbi.nlm.nih.gov/books/NBK536949/
5. Hadar, E., Ashwal, E., & Hod, M. (2015). The preconceptional period as an opportunity for prediction and prevention of noncommunicable disease. *Best Practice & Research Clinical Obstetrics & Gynaecology*, *29*(1), 54–62. https://doi.org/10.1016/j.bpobgyn.2014.05.011
6. Fuehrer, L., Buckler, E., Bowman, E., Gregory, T., & McDaniel, J. (2015). Promoting preconception health in primary care. *Journal of the American Academy of PAs*, *28*(8), 27–32. https://doi.org/10.1097/01.JAA.0000469436.52325.cb
7. Hurst, H. M., & Linton, D. M. (2015). Preconception care: Planning for the future. *The Journal for Nurse Practitioners*, *11*(3), 335–340. https://doi.org/10.1016/j.nurpra.2014.09.011
8. The American College of Obstetricians and Gynecologists (2024). *Good health before pregnancy: Prepregnancy care*. www.acog.org/womens-health/faqs/good-health-before-pregnancy-prepregnancy-care
9. D'Angelo, D. V., Bauman, B. L., Broussard, C. S., Tong, V. T., Ko, J. Y., Kapaya, M., Harrison, L., & Ahluwalia, I. B. (2019). Prevalence and maternal characteristics associated with receipt of prenatal care provider counseling about medications safe to take during pregnancy. *Preventive Medicine*, *126*, 105743. https://doi.org/10.1016/j.ypmed.2019.06.001
10. Gregory, E. F., Henry, D., & Akers, A. Y. (2021). Preconception and interconception pediatric primary care utilization of pregnant and parenting teens. *The Journal of Adolescent Health*, *69*(2), 315–320. https://doi.org/10.1016/j.jadohealth.2020.12.132
11. Interrante, J. D., & Flores, A. L. (2018). Discussing appropriate medication use and multivitamin intake with a healthcare provider: An examination of two elements of preconception care among Latinas. *Journal of Women's Health*, *27*(3), 348–358. https://doi.org/10.1089/jwh.2017.6421
12. Nobles-Botkin, J., Lincoln, A., & Cline, J. (2016). Preconception care resources: Where to start. *Journal of Midwifery & Women's Health*, *61*(3), 365–369. https://doi.org/10.1111/jmwh.12464
13. Kotelchuck, M., & Lu, M. (2017). Father's role in preconception health. *Maternal and Child Health Journal*, *21*(11), 2025–2039. https://doi.org/10.1007/s10995-017-2370-4
14. Mello, S., Stifano, S., Tan, A. S., Sanders-Jackson, A., & Bigman, C. A. (2020). Gendered conceptions of preconception health: A thematic analysis of men's and women's beliefs about responsibility for preconception health behavior. *Journal of Health Communication*, *25*(5), 374–384. https://doi.org/10.1080/10810730.2020.1775728

15. Thompson, E. L., Vázquez-Otero, C., Vamos, C. A., Marhefka, S. L., Kline, N. S., & Daley, E. M. (2017). Rethinking preconception care: A critical, women's health perspective. *Maternal and Child Health Journal*, *21*(5), 1147–1155. https://doi.org/10.1007/s10995-016-2213-8
16. Centers for Disease Control (2024, May 15). *Unintended pregnancy*. https://www.cdc.gov/reproductive-health/hcp/unintended-pregnancy/index.html
17. Dude, A. M., Schueler, K., Schumm, L. P., Murugesan, M., & Stulberg, D. B. (2022). Preconception care and severe maternal morbidity in the United States. *American Journal of Obstetrics & Gynecology MFM*, *4*(2), 100549. https://doi.org/10.1016/j.ajogmf.2021.100549
18. Horwitz, M. E. M., Ross-Degnan, D., & Pace, L. E. (2019). Contraceptive initiation among women in the United States: Timing, methods used, and pregnancy outcomes. *Pediatrics*, *143*(2). https://doi.org/10.1542/peds.2018-2463
19. Steinberg, J. R., Harrison, E. Y., & Boudreaux, M. (2020). Psychosocial factors associated with postpartum contraceptive method use after an unintended birth. *Obstetrics & Gynecology*, *135*(4), 821–831. https://doi.org/10.1097/AOG.0000000000003745
20. Gauthreaux, C., Negron, J., Castellanos, D., Ward-Peterson, M., Castro, G., de la Vega, P. R., & Acuña, J. M. (2017). The association between pregnancy intendedness and experiencing symptoms of postpartum depression among new mothers in the United States, 2009 to 2011: A secondary analysis of PRAMS data. *Medicine*, *96*(6). https://doi.org/10.1097/MD.0000000000005851
21. National Health Service (2024). *Sex and contraception after birth*. www.nhs.uk/conditions/baby/support-and-services/sex-and-contraception-after-birth/
22. The American College of Obstetricians and Gynecologists (2021). *Interpregnancy care*. www.acog.org/clinical/clinical-guidance/obstetric-care-consensus/articles/2019/01/interpregnancy-care#:~:text=.org%2Fbreastfeeding%20.-,Interpregnancy%20Interval,pregnancy%20sooner%20than%2018%20months
23. American College of Obstetricians and Gynecologists and the Society for Maternal-Fetal Medicine, Louis, J. M., Bryant, A., Ramos, D., Stuebe, A., & Blackwell, S. C. (2019). Interpregnancy care. *American Journal of Obstetrics & Gynecology*, *220*(1), PB2–B18. www.ajog.org/article/S0002-9378(18)32144-6/fulltext
24. Perin, J., & Walker, N. (2015). Potential confounding in the association between short birth intervals and increased neonatal, infant, and child mortality. *Global Health Action*, *8*, 29724. https://doi.org/10.3402/gha.v8.29724
25. Schummers, L., Hutcheon, J. A., Hernandez-Diaz, S., Williams, P. L., Hacker, M. R., VanderWeele, T. J., & Norman, W. V. (2018). Association of short interpregnancy interval with pregnancy outcomes according to maternal age. *JAMA Internal Medicine*, *178*(12), 1661–1670. https://doi.org/10.1001/jamainternmed.2018.4696
26. Thoma, M. E., De Silva, D. A., & MacDorman, M. F. (2019). Examining interpregnancy intervals and maternal and perinatal health outcomes using U.S. vital records: Important considerations for analysis and interpretation. *Paediatric and Perinatal Epidemiology*, *33*(1), O60–O72. https://doi.org/10.1111/ppe.12520
27. Yee, L. M., Truong, Y. N., Caughey, A. B., & Cheng, Y. W. (2016). The association between interdelivery interval and adverse perinatal outcomes in a diverse US population. *Journal of Perinatology*, *36*(8), 593–597. https://doi.org/10.1038/jp.2016.54
28. Garg, B., Darney, B., Pilliod, R. A., & Caughey, A. B. (2021). Long and short interpregnancy intervals increase severe maternal morbidity. *American Journal of Obstetrics and Gynecology*, *225*(3), 331.e1–331.e8. https://doi.org/10.1016/j.ajog.2021.05.013
29. Kangatharan, C., Labram, S., & Bhattacharya, S. (2017). Interpregnancy interval following miscarriage and adverse pregnancy outcomes: Systematic review and meta-analysis. *Human Reproduction Update*, *23*(2), 221–231. https://doi.org/10.1093/humupd/dmw043
30. Sundermann, A. C., Hartmann, K. E., Jones, S. H., Torstenson, E. S., & Edwards, D. R. V. (2017). Interpregnancy interval after pregnancy loss and risk of repeat miscarriage. *Obstetrics and Gynecology*, *130*(6), 1312. https://doi.org/10.1097/AOG.0000000000002318
31. Rutledge, R. I., Domino, M. E., Hillemeier, M. M., & Wells, R. (2016). The effect of maternity care coordination services on utilization of postpartum contraceptive services. *Contraception*, *94*(5), 541–547. https://doi.org/10.1016/j.contraception.2016.06.007
32. Lewin, A., Mitchell, S. J., Quinn, D. A., Street, T. M., Schmitz, K., & Beers, L. S. (2019). A primary care intervention to prevent repeat pregnancy among teen mothers. *American Journal of Preventive Medicine*, *56*(3), 404–410. https://doi.org/10.1016/j.amepre.2018.10.015

33. Coleman-Minahan, K., & Potter, J. E. (2019). Quality of postpartum contraceptive counseling and changes in contraceptive method preferences. *Contraception*, *100*(6), 492–497. https://doi.org/10.1016/j.contraception.2019.08.011
34. Toscano, M., Li, D., Dye, T., & Olson-Chen, C. (2019). Antepartum contraceptive counseling in women with preterm birth. *American Journal of Perinatology*, *36*(12), 1310–1316. https://doi.org/10.1055/s-0038-1676831
35. Lopez, L. M., Hiller, J. E., Grimes, D. A., & Chen, M. (2012). Education for contraceptive use by women after childbirth. *The Cochrane Database of Systematic Reviews*, *8*, CD001863. https://doi.org/10.1002/14651858.CD001863.pub3
36. Cha, S., Chapman, D. A., Wan, W., Burton, C. W., & Masho, S. W. (2016). Discordant pregnancy intentions in couples and rapid repeat pregnancy. *American Journal of Obstetrics and Gynecology*, *214*(4), 494-e1. https://doi.org/10.1016/j.ajog.2015.10.149
37. Shah, J. S., Revere, F. L., & Toy, E. C. (2018). Improving rates of early entry prenatal care in an underserved population. *Maternal and Child Health Journal*, *22*(12), 1738–1742. https://doi.org/10.1007/s10995-018-2569-z
38. American Academy of Pediatrics & The American College of Obstetricians and Gynecologists (2017). *Guidelines for perinatal care* (8th ed.). https://doi.org/10.1542/9781610020886
39. Osterman, M. J. K., & Martin, J. A. (2018, May). Timing and adequacy of prenatal care in the United States, 2016. *Statistics Reports*, *67*(3). www.cdc.gov/nchs/data/nvsr/nvsr67/nvsr67_03.pdf. Accessed December 2024.
40. Page, A., McCann, R., Maness, S., Merriweather, M., & Dobbs, P. D. (2024). Beyond the first trimester: Social determinants of delayed prenatal care at a community health center using the PRAPARE tool. *Journal of Racial and Ethnic Health Disparities*. https://doi.org/10.1007/s40615-024-02052-7. Advance online publication.
41. Simeone, R. M., Reefhuis, J., Jamieson, D. J., Drews-Botsch, C. D., Lash, T. L., Fisher, S. C., Howley, M. M., Evans, S., Howards, P. P., & National Birth Defects Prevention Study (2022). Delayed entry into prenatal care among women with pre-pregnancy health conditions, National Birth Defects Prevention Study, 1997–2011. *Preventive Medicine*, *164*, 107272. https://doi.org/10.1016/j.ypmed.2022.107272
42. Hacker, M., Firk, C., Konrad, K., Paschke, K., Neulen, J., Herpertz-Dahlmann, B., & Dahmen, B. (2021). Pregnancy complications, substance abuse, and prenatal care predict birthweight in adolescent mothers. *Archives of Public Health*, *79*(1), 137. https://doi.org/10.1186/s13690-021-00642-z
43. Gardner, M. E., Umer, A., Rudisill, T., Hendricks, B., Lefeber, C., John, C., & Lilly, C. (2023). Prenatal care and infant outcomes of teenage births: A Project WATCH study. *BMC Pregnancy and Childbirth*, *23*(1), 379. https://doi.org/10.1186/s12884-023-05662-x
44. Xaverius, P., Alman, C., Holtz, L., & Yarber, L. (2016). Risk factors associated with very low birth weight in a large urban area, stratified by adequacy of prenatal care. *Maternal and Child Health Journal*, *20*(3), 623–629. https://doi.org/10.1007/s10995-015-1861-4
45. Yan, J. (2017). The effects of prenatal care utilization on maternal health and health behaviors. *Health Economics*, *26*(8), 1001–1018. https://doi.org/10.1002/hec.3380
46. Dutra, G. R. S. D. F., Dutra, L. D. C., Fonsêca, G. K. S. D., Nascimento Júnior, M. B. D., & Lucena, E. E. D. S. (2018). Prenatal care and hypertensive gestational syndromes: A systematic review. *Revista Brasileira de Ginecologia e Obstetrícia*, *40*(8), 471–476. https://doi.org/10.1055/s-0038-1660526
47. Allen, A. J., Snowden, J. M., Lau, B., Cheng, Y., & Caughey, A. B. (2018). Type-2 diabetes mellitus: Does prenatal care affect outcomes? *The Journal of Maternal-Fetal & Neonatal Medicine*, *31*(1), 93–97. https://doi.org/10.1080/14767058.2016.1276558
48. ACOG Committee Opinion (2017, September). *Update on immunization and pregnancy tetanus diptheria and pertussis vaccination*. www.acog.org/-/media/project/acog/acogorg/clinical/files/committee-opinion/articles/2017/09/update-on-immunization-and-pregnancy-tetanus-diphtheria-and-pertussis-vaccination.pdf
49. ACOG Committee Opinion (2018, April). *Influenza vaccination during pregnancy*. www.acog.org/-/media/project/acog/acogorg/clinical/files/committee-opinion/articles/2018/04/influenza-vaccination-during-pregnancy.pdf

50. ACOG Committee Opinion (2018, June). *Maternal immunization.* www.acog.org/-/media/project/acog/acogorg/clinical/files/committee-opinion/articles/2018/06/maternal-immunization.pdf
51. ACOG (2020, December). *COVID-19 vaccination considerations for obstetric gynecologic care.* www.acog.org/clinical/clinical-guidance/practice-advisory/articles/2020/12/covid-19-vaccination-considerations-for-obstetric-gynecologic-care
52. The American College of Obstetricians and Gynecologists (2024). *Vaccines during pregnancy.* www.acog.org/womens-health/infographics/vaccines-during-pregnancy
53. Getahun, D., Fassett, M. J., Peltier, M. R., Takhar, H. S., Shaw, S. F., Im, T. M., Chiu, V. Y., & Jacobsen, S. J. (2019). Association between seasonal influenza vaccination with pre-and postnatal outcomes. *Vaccine, 37*(13), 1785–1791. https://doi.org/10.1016/j.vaccine.2019.02.019
54. Zerbo, O., Modaressi, S., Chan, B., Goddard, K., Lewis, N., Bok, K., Fireman, B., Klein, N., & Baxter, R. (2017). No association between influenza vaccination during pregnancy and adverse birth outcomes. *Vaccine, 35*(24), 3186–3190. https://doi.org/10.1016/j.vaccine.2017.04.074
55. Madhi, S. A., & Nunes, M. C. (2018). Experience and challenges on influenza and pertussis vaccination in pregnant women. *Human Vaccines & Immunotherapeutics, 14*(9), 2183–2188. https://doi.org/10.1080/21645515.2018.1483810
56. Chan, H. J., Chang, J. Y., Erickson, S. R., & Wang, C. C. (2019). Influenza vaccination among pregnant women in the United States: Findings from the 2012–2016 National Health Interview Survey. *Journal of Women's Health, 28*(7), 965–975. https://doi.org/10.1089/jwh.2018.7139
57. Ding, H., Kahn, K. E., Black, C. L., O'Halloran, A., Lu, P. J., & Williams, W. W. (2019). Influenza vaccination coverage among pregnant women in the US, 2012–2015. *American Journal of Preventive Medicine, 56*(4), 477–486. https://doi.org/10.1016/j.amepre.2018.11.020
58. O'Leary, S. T., Pyrzanowski, J., Brewer, S. E., Barnard, J., Beaty, B., Donnelly, M., Mazzoni, S., & Dempsey, A. F. (2015). Influenza and pertussis vaccination among pregnant women and their infants' close contacts: Reported practices and attitudes. *The Pediatric Infectious Disease Journal, 34*(11), 1244–1249. https://doi.org/10.1097/INF.0000000000000873
59. Etti, M., Calvert, A., Galiza, E., Lim, S., Khalil, A., Le Doare, K., & Heath, P. T. (2022). Maternal vaccination: A review of current evidence and recommendations. *American Journal of Obstetrics and Gynecology, 226*(4), 459–474. https://doi.org/10.1016/j.ajog.2021.10.041
60. Triunfo, S., Iannuzzi, V., Podda, M., Pedrina, D., Gemelli, S., & Marconi, A. M. (2023). Reducing vaccine hesitancy in pregnancy by the health literacy model inclusive of modern communication tools. *Archives of Gynecology and Obstetrics, 308*(5), 1391–1393. https://doi.org/10.1007/s00404-023-07138-x
61. Lindley, M. C., Kahn, K. E., Bardenheier, B. H., D'Angelo, D. V., Dawood, F. S., Fink, R. V., Havers, F., & Skoff, T. H. (2019). Vital signs: Burden and prevention of influenza and pertussis among pregnant women and infants – United States. *Morbidity and Mortality Weekly Report, 68*(40), 885. https://doi.org/10.15585/mmwr.mm6840e1. Accessed December 2024.
62. Henninger, M. L., Irving, S. A., Thompson, M., Avalos, L. A., Ball, S. W., Shifflett, P., Naleway, A. L., & Pregnancy and Influenza Project (PIP) Working Group (2015). Factors associated with seasonal influenza vaccination in pregnant women. *Journal of Women's Health, 24*(5), 394–402. https://doi.org/10.1089/jwh.2014.5105
63. Wales, D. P., Khan, S., Suresh, D., Ata, A., & Morris, B. (2020). Factors associated with Tdap vaccination receipt during pregnancy: A cross-sectional study. *Public Health, 179*, 38–44. https://doi.org/10.1016/j.puhe.2019.10.001
64. Bushar, J. A., Kendrick, J. S., Ding, H., Black, C. L., & Greby, S. M. (2017). Text4baby influenza messaging and influenza vaccination among pregnant women. *American Journal of Preventive Medicine, 53*(6), 845–853. https://doi.org/10.1016/j.amepre.2017.06.021
65. Jordan, E. T., Bushar, J. A., Kendrick, J. S., Johnson, P., & Wang, J. (2015). Encouraging influenza vaccination among Text4baby pregnant women and mothers. *American Journal of Preventive Medicine, 49*(4), 563–572. https://doi.org/10.1016/j.amepre.2015.04.029
66. O'Leary, S. T., Narwaney, K. J., Wagner, N. M., Kraus, C. R., Omer, S. B., & Glanz, J. M. (2019). Efficacy of a web-based intervention to increase uptake of maternal vaccines: An RCT.

American Journal of Preventive Medicine, *57*(4), e125–e133. https://doi.org/10.1016/j.amepre.2019.05.018

67. The American College of Obstetricians and Gynecologists (2022). *Oral health care during pregnancy and through the lifespan*. www.acog.org/clinical/clinical-guidance/committee-opinion/articles/2013/08/oral-health-care-during-pregnancy-and-through-the-lifespan
68. Umer, A., Haile, Z. T., Ahmadi-Montecalvo, H., & Chertok, I. R. (2016). Factors associated with receipt of pre-pregnancy preventive dental care among women in West Virginia: Pregnancy risk assessment monitoring system (PRAMS) survey 2009–2010. *Oral Health & Preventive Dentistry*, *14*(5), 413–422. https://doi.org/10.3290/j.ohpd.a36467
69. Silveira, M. L., Whitcomb, B. W., Pekow, P., Carbone, E. T., & Chasan-Taber, L. (2016). Anxiety, depression, and oral health among US pregnant women: 2010 Behavioral Risk Factor Surveillance System. *Journal of Public Health Dentistry*, *76*(1), 56–64. https://doi.org/10.1111/jphd.12112
70. Fryer, K., Munoz, M. C., Rahangdale, L., & Stuebe, A. M. (2021). Multiparous Black and Latinx women face more barriers to prenatal care than White women. *Journal of Racial and Ethnic Health Disparities*, *8*(1), 80–87. https://doi.org/10.1007/s40615-020-00759-x
71. Peahl, A. F., Pennathur, H., Zacharek, N., Naccarato, A., Heberle-Rose, H., Goodman, J., Smith, R. D., Cohn, A., Stout, M. J., Fendrick, A. M., & Moniz, M. H. (2024). Retrospective use of patients' characteristics to assess variation in prenatal care utilization. *American Journal of Perinatology*, *41*(S 01), e2529–e2538. https://doi.org/10.1055/s-0043-1771505
72. Baer, R. J., Altman, M. R., Oltman, S. P., Ryckman, K. K., Chambers, C. D., Rand, L., & Jelliffe-Pawlowski, L. L. (2019). Maternal factors influencing late entry into prenatal care: A stratified analysis by race or ethnicity and insurance status. *The Journal of Maternal-Fetal & Neonatal Medicine*, *32*(20), 3336–3342. https://doi.org/10.1080/14767058.2018.1463366
73. Kentoffio, K., Berkowitz, S. A., Atlas, S. J., Oo, S. A., & Percac-Lima, S. (2016). Use of maternal health services: Comparing refugee, immigrant and US-born populations. *Maternal and Child Health Journal*, *20*(12), 2494–2501. https://doi.org/10.1007/s10995-016-2072-3
74. Garcia, K. K., & Hunter, S. K. (2022). Proposed solutions for improving maternal health care in rural America. *Clinical Obstetrics and Gynecology*, *65*(4), 868–876. https://doi.org/10.1097/GRF.0000000000000754
75. Habtemariam, H., Schlichting, L. E., Kole-White, M. B., Berger, B., & Vivier, P. (2024). Neighborhood risk and prenatal care utilization in Rhode Island, 2005–2014. *Birth*, *51*(3), 559–570. https://doi.org/10.1111/birt.12810
76. Mager, N. A. D., Zollinger, T. W., Turman, J. E., Jr., Zhang, J., & Dixon, B. E. (2021). Routine healthcare utilization among reproductive-age women residing in a rural maternity care desert. *Journal of Community Health*, *46*(1), 108–116. https://doi.org/10.1007/s10900-020-00852-6
77. Hung, P., Casey, M. M., Kozhimannil, K. B., Karaca-Mandic, P., & Moscovice, I. S. (2018). Rural-urban differences in access to hospital obstetric and neonatal care: How far is the closest one? *Journal of Perinatology*, *38*(6), 645–652. https://doi.org/10.1038/s41372-018-0063-5
78. Hung, P., Henning-Smith, C. E., Casey, M. M., & Kozhimannil, K. B. (2017). Access to obstetric services in rural counties still declining, with 9 percent losing services, 2004–14. *Health Affairs*, *36*(9), 1663–1671. https://doi.org/10.1377/hlthaff.2017.0338
79. Mitra, M., Parish, S. L., Clements, K. M., Cui, X., & Diop, H. (2015). Pregnancy outcomes among women with intellectual and developmental disabilities. *American Journal of Preventive Medicine*, *48*(3), 300–308. https://doi.org/10.1016/j.amepre.2014.09.032
80. Mitra, M., Akobirshoev, I., Moring, N. S., Long-Bellil, L., Smeltzer, S. C., Smith, L. D., & Iezzoni, L. I. (2017). Access to and satisfaction with prenatal care among pregnant women with physical disabilities: Findings from a national survey. *Journal of Women's Health*, *26*(12), 1356–1363. https://doi.org/10.1089/jwh.2016.6297
81. Cunningham, S. D., Magriples, U., Thomas, J. L., Kozhimannil, K. B., Herrera, C., Barrette, E., Shebl, F. M., & Ickovics, J. R. (2017). Association between maternal comorbidities and emergency department use among a national sample of commercially insured pregnant women. *Academic Emergency Medicine*, *24*(8), 940–947. https://doi.org/10.1111/acem.13215
82. Malik, S., Kothari, C., MacCallum, C., Liepman, M., Tareen, S., & Rhodes, K. V. (2017). Emergency department use in the perinatal period: An opportunity for early intervention. *Annals of Emergency Medicine*, *70*(6), 835–839. https://doi.org/10.1016/j.annemergmed.2017.06.020

83. Mehta, P. K., Carter, T., Vinoya, C., Kangovi, S., & Srinivas, S. K. (2017). Understanding high utilization of unscheduled care in pregnant women of low socioeconomic status. *Women's Health Issues*, *27*(4), 441–448. https://doi.org/10.1016/j.whi.2017.01.007
84. Nijagal, M. A., Patel, D., Lyles, C., Liao, J., Chehab, L., Williams, S., & Sammann, A. (2021). Using human-centered design to identify opportunities for reducing inequities in perinatal care. *BMC Health Services Research*, *21*(714). https://doi.org/10.1186/s12913-021-06609-8
85. Thai, A., & Johnson, K. M. (2022). Relationship between perceived quality of prenatal care and maternal/infant health outcomes. *Southern Medical Journal*, *115*(12), 893–898. https://doi.org/10.14423/SMJ.0000000000001483
86. ACOG Committee Opinion No. 587: Effective patient-physician communication. (2014). *Obstetrics and Gynecology*, *123*(2 Pt 1), 389–393. https://doi.org/10.1097/01.AOG.0000443279.14017.12
87. Berk, A. L., Pickett, A., Kusters, I. S., & Gregory, M. E. (2024). Healthcare experiences of Black patients during and after pregnancy: A needs assessment for provider training to improve quality of care. *Journal of Racial and Ethnic Health Disparities*, *11*(2), 992–1004. https://doi.org/10.1007/s40615-023-01579-5
88. Louis, M. S., Mangal, R. K., Stead, T. S., Jones, T., & Ganti, L. (2023). Racial disparities in satisfaction with maternal healthcare. *Journal of the National Medical Association*, *115*(6), 589–592. https://doi.org/10.1016/j.jnma.2023.10.001
89. Mohamoud, Y. A., Cassidy, E., Fuchs, E., Womack, L. S., Romero, L., Kipling, L., Oza-Frank, R., Baca, K., Galang, R. R., Stewart, A., Carrigan, S., Mullen, J., Busacker, A., Behm, B., Hollier, L. M., Kroelinger, C., Mueller, T., Barfield, W. D., & Cox, S. (2023). Vital signs: Maternity care experiences – United States, April 2023. *MMWR. Morbidity and Mortality Weekly Report*, *72*(35), 961–967. https://doi.org/10.15585/mmwr.mm7235e1. Accessed December 2024.
90. Murphy, L., & Liu, F. (2022). A new perspective on the maternal mortality disparity. *Nursing Forum*, *57*(1), 171–176. https://doi.org/10.1111/nuf.12652
91. Prater, C., Cohen, L., Chau, E., Carter, E. B., Kuebee, B., Tepe, M., & Keegan, M. (2023). Perceived discrimination during prenatal care at a community health center. *Journal of Racial and Ethnic Health Disparities*, *10*(3), 1304–1309. https://doi.org/10.1007/s40615-022-01315-5
92. Ward, T. C. S., Mazul, M., Ngui, E. M., Bridgewater, F. D., & Harley, A. E. (2013). "You learn to go last": Perceptions of prenatal care experiences among African-American women with limited incomes. *Maternal and Child Health Journal*, *17*(10), 1753–1759. https://doi.org/10.1007/s10995-012-1194-5
93. Weber, A., Miskle, B., Lynch, A., Arndt, S., & Acion, L. (2021). Substance use in pregnancy: Identifying stigma and improving care. *Substance Abuse and Rehabilitation*, *12*, 105–121. https://doi.org/10.2147/SAR.S319180
94. Goh, A. H., Altman, M. R., Canty, L., & Edmonds, J. K. (2024). Communication between pregnant people of color and prenatal care providers in the United States: An integrative review. *Journal of Midwifery & Women's Health*, *69*(2), 202–223. https://doi.org/10.1111/jmwh.13580
95. Coley, S. L., Zapata, J. Y., Schwei, R. J., Mihalovic, G. E., Matabele, M. N., Jacobs, E. A., & Anderson, C. K. (2018). More than a "number": Perspectives of prenatal care quality from mothers of color and providers. *Women's Health Issues*, *28*(2), 158–164. https://doi.org/10.1016/j.whi.2017.10.014
96. Evans, N. M., & Sheu, J. (2019). Validating a path model of adherence to prenatal care recommendations among pregnant women. *Patient Education and Counseling*, *102*, 1350–1356. https://doi.org/10.1016/j.pec.2019.02.028
97. Schmuke, A. D. (2019). Factors affecting uncertainty in women with high-risk pregnancies. *MCN: The American Journal of Maternal/Child Nursing*, *44*(6), 317–324. https://doi.org/10.1097/NMC.0000000000000563
98. Adams, C., & Thomas, S. P. (2017). Alternative prenatal care interventions to alleviate Black–White maternal/infant health disparities. *Sociology Compass*, *12*(1), e12549. https://doi.org/10.1111/soc4.12549
99. Heberlein, E. C., Picklesimer, A. H., Billings, D. L., Covington-Kolb, S., Farber, N., & Frongillo, E. A. (2016). The comparative effects of group prenatal care on psychosocial

outcomes. *Archives of Women's Mental Health, 19*(2), 259–269. https://doi.org/10.1007/s00737-015-0564-6

100. Keller, J. M., Norton, J. A., Zhang, F., Paul, R., Madden, T., Raghuraman, N., Stout, M. J., & Carter, E. B. (2023). The impact of group prenatal care on interpregnancy interval. *American Journal of Perinatology, 40*(15), 1659–1664. https://doi.org/10.1055/s-0041-1739413
101. Tubay, A. T., Mansalis, K. A., Simpson, M. J., Armitage, N. H., Briscoe, G., & Potts, V. (2019). The effects of group prenatal care on infant birthweight and maternal well-being: A randomized controlled trial. *Military Medicine, 184*(5–6), e440–e446. https://doi.org/10.1093/milmed/usy361
102. McCue, B. K., & Borders, A. E. (2018). Group prenatal care. *Obstetrics and Gynecology, 131*(3), E104–E108. https://doi.org/10.1097/AOG.0000000000002529
103. Heberlein, E. C., Picklesimer, A. H., Billings, D. L., Covington-Kolb, S., Farber, N., & Frongillo, E. A. (2016). Qualitative comparison of women's perspectives on the functions and benefits of group and individual prenatal care. *Journal of Midwifery & Women's Health, 61*(2), 224–234. https://doi.org/10.1111/jmwh.12379
104. Byerley, B. M., & Haas, D. M. (2017). A systematic overview of the literature regarding group prenatal care for high-risk pregnant women. *BMC Pregnancy and Childbirth, 17*(1), 1–9. https://doi.org/10.1186/s12884-017-1522-2
105. Augur, M., Ellis, S. A., & Moon, J. (2022). The Early Care Model for initiation of perinatal care: "I actually felt listened to." *Journal of Midwifery & Women's Health, 67*(6), 735–739. https://doi.org/10.1111/jmwh.13435
106. Weisband, Y. L., Gallo, M. F., Klebanoff, M., Shoben, A., & Norris, A. H. (2018). Who uses a midwife for prenatal care and for birth in the United States? A secondary analysis of Listening to Mothers III. *Women's Health Issues, 28*(1), 89–96. https://doi.org/10.1016/j.whi.2017.07.004
107. Turienzo, C. F., Sandall, J., & Peacock, J. L. (2016). Models of antenatal care to reduce and prevent preterm birth: A systematic review and meta-analysis. *BMJ Open, 6*(1). https://doi.org/0.1136/bmjopen-2015-009044
108. Weisband, Y. L., Gallo, M. F., Klebanoff, M. A., Shoben, A. B., & Norris, A. H. (2018). Progression of care among women who use a midwife for prenatal care: Who remains in midwife care? *Birth, 45*(1), 28–36. https://doi.org/10.1111/birt.12308
109. Kern-Goldberger, A., & Hirshberg, A. (2021). Reducing disparities using telehealth approaches for postdelivery preeclampsia care. *Clinical Obstetrics and Gynecology, 64*(2), 375–383. https://doi.org/10.1097/GRF.0000000000000605
110. The American College of Obstetricians and Gynecologists (2020). *Implementing telehealth in practice.* www.acog.org/clinical/clinical-guidance/committee-opinion/articles/2020/02/implementing-telehealth-in-practice
111. Aziz, A., Zork, N., Aubey, J. J., Baptiste, C. D., D'Alton, M. E., Emeruwa, U. N., Fuchs, K., Goffman, D., Gyamfi-Bannerman, C., Haythe, J. H., LaSala, A. P., Madden, N., Miller, E. C., Miller, R. S., Monk, C., Moroz, L., Ona, S., Ring, L. E., Sheen, J. J., Spiegel, E. S., Simpsnoe, L. L., Yates, H. S., & Friedman, A. M. (2020). Telehealth for high-risk pregnancies in the setting of the COVID-19 pandemic. *American Journal of Perinatology, 37*(8), 800. https://doi.org/10.1055/s-0040-1712121
112. Bruno, B., Mercer, M. B., Hizlan, S., Peskin, J., Ford, P. J., Farrell, R. M., & Rose, S. L. (2023). Virtual prenatal visits associated with high measures of patient experience and satisfaction among average-risk patients: A prospective cohort study. *BMC Pregnancy and Childbirth, 23*(1), 234. https://doi.org/10.1186/s12884-023-05421-y
113. Peahl, A. F., Smith, R. D., & Moniz, M. H. (2020). Prenatal care redesign: Creating flexible maternity care models through virtual care. *American Journal of Obstetrics and Gynecology, 223*(3), 389.e1–389.e10. https://doi.org/10.1016/j.ajog.2020.05.029
114. Lee, J., & Manalew, W. S. (2023). Reasons for not pursuing virtual prenatal care in 2020 through 2021 and policy implications. *Telemedicine Journal and E-Health: The Official Journal of the American Telemedicine Association, 29*(10), 1492–1503. https://doi.org/10.1089/tmj.2022.0492

7 Healthcare During Childbirth and the Postpartum Period

Self-Care Moment

During pregnancy and the postpartum period, patients are often encouraged to stay well hydrated, particularly if they are breastfeeding or have a health condition like gestational diabetes. Once again, it is important for us to "walk the talk" around any advice that we give. When was the last time you had a glass of water? If it has been a while, grab one before continuing with this chapter.

High-quality, culturally sensitive healthcare is essential to ensuring maternal and infant health and safety in the year following childbirth. When such care is not accessible, there is an increased risk of health problems/complications – and even death. Therefore, in recent years, numerous trainings and resources have been developed for healthcare providers with the hope of improving the quality and cultural sensitivity of care that they provide to their pregnant and postpartum patients.

This chapter takes a different approach by focusing on issues related to health and healthcare during childbirth and the postpartum period that are important for community and social service providers to know about. Community and social service providers who know about these issues are well positioned to help their clients navigate healthcare options, advocate for themselves, and have their voices heard. Content in this chapter includes discussion of research on this topic, practice implications for your work, and reflections on your role as a community or social service provider. You will also hear the stories of Kimberly Turbin, a survivor of obstetric violence; Chen and Katie, who experienced bias as an LGBTQ+ couple during childbirth; and Tatiana, who had the experience of feeling unheard and unsupported during postpartum care.

Key Terms

Cesarean section (or C-section, or Cesarean birth): The surgical delivery of a baby through an incision in the abdomen and uterus.

Labor induction (or induction of labor): A procedure that uses drugs or other medical methods to start labor.

Elective induction: Labor induction that is initiated for non-medical reasons before the body goes into labor on its own (typically close to one's due date).

DOI: 10.4324/9781003476474-7

Interprofessional care: A collaborative approach to healthcare in which professionals from different disciplines work together to provide comprehensive, coordinated, and patient-centered care.

Out-of-hospital birth: Childbirth that occurs outside a hospital setting; for example, at home or at a community birth center.

Unattended birth (sometimes called "free birth"): Childbirth that occurs without a healthcare professional in attendance.

Doula: A non-medical professional who has been trained to provide support, education, and advocacy during pregnancy, childbirth, and/or the postpartum period.

Research Summary

Relationships With Healthcare and Childbirth Professionals and Medical Bias

Self-Care Moment

The paragraph below tells the story of Kimberly Turbin, a woman who experienced obstetric violence during childbirth. We feel that it is important to share her story as an example of what too many individuals – particularly people of color – experience. However, we encourage you to take care of yourself. If needed, you can skip to the main text below Kimberly's story.

Kimberly's Story ∞

Kimberly Turbin, a Latina from Los Angeles, California, has widely shared her story of mistreatment during the birth of her son, including a YouTube video of the birth. Before giving birth, Kimberly let her obstetrician know that she was a survivor of multiple sexual assaults. She asked him to be as gentle as possible and to keep her informed throughout the childbirth process. Despite this, as well as the fact that neither Kimberly nor her baby was experiencing medical distress, and that leading medical organizations urge that episiotomies should only be conducted when truly necessary, her doctor conducted an episiotomy – making numerous cuts to her perineum (the area between the vagina and anus). In the childbirth video taken by her mother, Kimberly can be heard saying "No!" many times. She went on to sue the doctor for assault and battery, and the doctor ultimately surrendered his medical license. Kimberly is now an advocate for respectful and sensitive care during pregnancy, and for survivors of obstetric violence.[1,2,3]

It is important that individuals feel supported, informed, and involved in decision-making about their healthcare throughout the entire childbirth process.[4] Preferences for who someone would like to receive support from (i.e., from a healthcare professional, doula, midwife, and/or loved one) may vary depending on their specific situation, cultural beliefs and values, and relationships.[5] However, research has found that the quality and amount of support provided by healthcare and childbirth professionals (i.e., obstetricians/gynecologists, midwives, nurses, doulas) has a large impact on how people feel about their birthing experience.[6] Relationships with healthcare and childbirth professionals have also been linked to both maternal and infant health outcomes.[7]

Unfortunately, many patients like Kimberly feel unsupported, unheard, and even mistreated by the healthcare and birthing professionals who are supposed to take care of them.[8,9,10,11] A multi-year study of first-time mothers in Pennsylvania found that women who were Black, who did not have a college degree, and who did not have private insurance were less likely to report that their provider kept them informed and involved in the decision-making process around childbirth – even in situations involving unplanned or complex interventions, such as labor induction, instrument-assisted vaginal delivery (i.e., with vacuum or forceps), or C-section.[12] Research has also found that patients of color may be more likely to undergo procedures (i.e., episiotomy, induction) during childbirth without their consent.[13] In another study, postpartum women of color commonly reported that their healthcare providers withheld or obscured information from them, creating a power dynamic that compromised their autonomy and ability to make informed healthcare decisions for themselves and their babies.[14]

Another study found that 28% of women who gave birth in a hospital reported mistreatment (i.e., being shouted at, scolded, threatened, or refused help), compared to only 5% of those with out-of-hospital births.[15] Women with lower socioeconomic resources, women of color, and those who needed unexpected interventions were more likely to report mistreatment.[15] On the other hand, White women, those with vaginal deliveries, those over the age of 30, those with previous childbirths, and those being treated by midwives were less likely to report mistreatment.[15]

The negative childbirth experiences of many patients of color are related to racism and implicit bias among healthcare and childbirth professionals. In a study of Black mothers in Texas, researchers found evidence of unbalanced patient–provider power dynamics across all childbirth settings (i.e., hospitals, community birth centers, attended home births). However, they found that use of overt domination and subordination techniques was more common in hospital settings.[16] In another study, many Black women reported receiving substandard and biased healthcare during childbirth, and that their healthcare providers responded poorly when they asked questions. The same women talked about how important it is for patients, particularly people of color, to have knowledgeable support people to help them navigate the healthcare system.[17] Participants in another study shared numerous recommendations for systems-level interventions that might improve the childbirth experiences of people of color (i.e., having the same provider throughout pregnancy and childbirth, matching patients to providers from similar racial or ethnic backgrounds, implicit bias trainings for healthcare and childbirth professionals).[14]

Several other groups also commonly report challenges and biases in their relationships with healthcare and childbirth professionals. One review found that immigrants in the United States often experience discrimination and communication barriers when giving birth, and that this group sometimes pursues out-of-hospital births due to fears of legal action or deportation.[18] Another group that has been repeatedly found to experience biased or insensitive treatment during birth are those who identify as LGBTQ+ and their families – pointing to the need for greater supports specific to LGBTQ+ health ne eds.[19,20,21,22]

Chen and Katie's Story ♥

When Chen gave birth to her first child, her wife Katie never left her side. However, throughout the couple's time at the hospital, they repeatedly experienced bias as an LGBTQ+ couple – adding significant stress to what should have been a joyful time. Chen and Katie were asked several times "where the baby's father was," and several people assumed they were sisters before learning they were married. When the family moved to the postpartum unit, their assigned nurse said that she was going to hand them off to a coworker because she "did not feel comfortable" working with them. This was the final straw that led Chen to burst into tears. "I just want to be treated with respect like everyone else," she said to Katie. "Is that too much to ask?"

Putting It Into Practice

- ***Be knowledgeable about culturally responsive healthcare providers in your local area.*** You can take note of clients' experiences with different healthcare providers and develop a personal or organizational "database" of capable, culturally sensitive local healthcare providers. You can share this information with families as they choose among different healthcare providers in their area, particularly if they are struggling with a current provider or are hesitant to get care for personal or cultural reasons.
- ***Support health literacy.*** The importance of feeling informed and involved in the healthcare decision-making process only increases over the course of pregnancy. Growing anxiety and excitement can also affect people's ability to remember information. As a community or social service provider, you can help your clients to process health information and guidance that they receive from their healthcare providers, focusing on key points and takeaways.
- ***Validate concerns.*** As a trusted professional in your clients' lives, you can validate their feelings and concerns about many things, including their experiences with healthcare providers. This validation can help individuals feel empowered to bring issues forward to their healthcare provider – and others in their healthcare system – as needed. You can also affirm when parents seem to be encountering biases and barriers, working with them to find alternative options while also seeking to address these issues at the systems level.

Take Time to Reflect

Think about any stories you have heard from clients, loved ones, or the media about experiencing mistreatment and/or medical bias during childbirth. What emotions do you feel as you remember those stories? In what ways do you think a community or social service provider like yourself could make a difference in a similar situation?

Childbirth Interventions and Settings

The next section of this chapter describes several key childbirth interventions and settings that community and social service providers should know about, including: (a) labor induction;

(b) C-section; (c) interprofessional care during hospital births; and (d) out-of-hospital births, including home births and births occurring at community birth centers.

Labor Induction

Nearly one-quarter of births in the United States involve labor induction.[23] Healthcare professionals typically recommend labor induction when a pregnancy reaches 41 weeks gestation, or when there are increasing or high-risk health problems/complications.[24] In these cases, labor induction is often an important step to protect both maternal and infant health and well-being.

Some individuals request elective inductions for non-medical reasons – for example, because they live far from away from a hospital and are afraid that if they go into labor naturally, they may not make it there in time; because they want the baby to be born within a specific time range; or because they are having a difficult last trimester and do not want to be pregnant any longer. Elective inductions are typically not recommended before 39 weeks gestation, as earlier inductions have been linked to increased health risks for babies.[25] There is mixed evidence about the health outcomes related to elective inductions conducted at 39 or 40 weeks gestation – some studies find no negative effects on maternal and infant health; others have found evidence of some increased risk.[26,27] Therefore, it is important that those who are interested in elective induction thoroughly discuss their individual situation and the potential risks and benefits with their healthcare provider.

Cesarean Sections

The rate of C-sections has risen in recent decades. For example, in the United States, the rate of C-sections rapidly increased between 1996 and 2011 to a rate of 1 of 3 live births, where it currently remains.[28] C-sections are essential and often life-saving procedures for situations when vaginal delivery is not safe or possible. This includes situations in which C-sections are planned in advance for medical reasons (i.e., when baby has been breech for several weeks), as well as situations in which C-sections are unplanned or conducted on an emergency basis (i.e., due to sudden health problems/complications during labor). C-sections can also be conducted on an elective basis for non-medical reasons (i.e., when someone prefers not to give birth vaginally for any number of reasons; also known as *Cesarean delivery on maternal request*).[29]

While a C-section can be an appropriate and life-saving option, it is important to keep in mind that it is major abdominal surgery. As such, it requires significant recovery time and it carries risk of health problems/complications for both the parent (i.e., cardiac arrest, acute renal failure, sepsis, death) and baby (i.e., breathing problems, increased chances of needing neonatal intensive care).[30,31,32] The reasons behind a C-section are important when it comes to risk and recovery. Research indicates that those who undergo emergency C-sections, as well as their babies, are more likely to experience health problems/complications or death than those who undergo elective C-sections.[33] Meanwhile, other work has shown that those with planned C-sections experience higher rates of complications and death than those with planned vaginal deliveries.[30] C-sections are also associated with increased risk of health problems/complications and additional C-sections in subsequent pregnancies.[34] As such, the American College of Obstetricians and Gynecologists and other groups advise that C-sections should be reserved for situations when vaginal delivery would carry significant health risks.[29] They also advise that voluntary C-sections should be conducted on a very limited basis in consideration of the patient's unique circumstances and medical needs.[29]

Research also suggests that certain groups are more likely to receive C-sections than others – for example, those who are over age 50, those who are delivering multiples, those undergoing elective induction, those with prior histories of uterine surgery or C-section, and/or those with cardiometabolic risk factors (i.e., obesity, diabetes).[35,36,37] Studies have also found higher cluster rates of C-sections in regions that are rural, that have fewer midwives, and that have high proportions of public insurance recipients.[38] Other work has found evidence of racial and ethnic disparities in C-section rates.[39,40,41,42,43,44] One study reported that Black individuals were more likely to have C-sections and to have long hospital stays compared to their White counterparts – a pattern which was evident across socioeconomic groups and insurance types.[45] Another study found that Black and Hispanic women with high BMIs were more likely to receive C-sections than White women with high BMIs.[46] These and other findings suggest that in some groups, heightened C-section rates may reflect true medical needs; but in others, heightened C-section rates likely reflect disparities in the quality of healthcare and support that certain groups receive during pregnancy and childbirth.

Take Time to Reflect

C-section rates vary widely across hospitals. This can sometimes be because certain hospitals serve greater numbers of high-risk patients; however, it can also be related to other factors at the hospital level, including medical bias. Write down the names of the hospitals that your clients most commonly give birth at. Now, open an online search engine and type: "[HOSPITAL NAME] C-section rates." See what information you can find and think about how it aligns or differs from the experiences of clients you have worked with.

Putting It Into Practice

- ***Help clients to reflect on their childbirth preferences.*** It is beneficial for people to go into childbirth with a good understanding of common childbirth interventions and how they feel about them. For some, this topic may be weighted with emotion due to their own prior experiences or the experiences of loved ones. These individuals may feel most comfortable and able to explore information about childbirth interventions within the context of the trusting relationship they have with you. Additionally, because you likely have more time to spend with families than their healthcare providers, they can explore information with you at a more relaxed pace.
- ***Help clients to decide who they would (and would not) like to support them during childbirth.*** Most individuals benefit from having a supportive person (or people) alongside them during the childbirth process to back them up, to speak up for them when they cannot do so, and to help ensure that the care they receive is respectful, safe, and high-quality. This support person can be a partner, family member or friend, doula (see discussion later in this chapter), or another trusted individual. For some people, it may also be important to discuss any people that they do not want present at the childbirth or in the waiting room, and how to plan for this.
- ***Support the development of a birth plan.*** It can be helpful to create a written birth plan that communicates one's preferences and desires for childbirth. You can

assist families by helping them locate and even complete a birth plan template. It is important to acknowledge that communicating their wishes in advance to their healthcare provider does not guarantee that non-preferred interventions/practices will not be used. Hopefully, however, a birth plan will increase the chances that non-preferred interventions/practices will only be used if absolutely necessary.

Interprofessional Care During Hospital Births

Research has found that in low-risk pregnancies, having an interprofessional care team (i.e., one that includes both a midwife and an obstetrician/gynecologist) is associated with lower C-section rates, lower rates of intervention (i.e., labor induction, oxytocin augmentation), and increased rates of vaginal birth in subsequent pregnancies.[47,48] The American College of Obstetricians and Gynecologists has also stated that collaboration between healthcare and childbirth professionals (i.e., obstetricians/gynecologists, midwives, nurses, doulas) is important for reducing unnecessary interventions and ensuring that patients feel informed and involved in the decision-making process.[49,50]

Out-of-Hospital Births

More and more individuals are choosing to give birth in settings outside of hospitals – for example, at home or at a community birth center. National data from the United States indicates that, between 2004 and 2017, the rate of home births increased by 77% and the rate of births occurring at community birth centers increased by 100%, with one out of every 62 births (1%) taking place outside of a hospital by 2017. The same study found that out-of-hospital births were most common in Pacific Northwest states. Those living in Southeastern states, adolescents, smokers, and those whose weight was in the obese range were less likely to have out-of-hospital births. Individuals with out-of-hospital births were also much more likely to self-pay than those who gave birth in a hospital. Specifically, 2 of 3 people (67%) who had a planned home birth and 1 of 3 people (33%) who gave birth at a community birth center paid the bill themselves, compared to 1 of 100 people (1%) who had a hospital birth.[51] Other evidence has indicated that, in the United States, out-of-hospital births are on the rise in rural areas, where many hospitals providing obstetric care have closed.[52]

A literature review on home births found that some of the reasons Americans choose home births include believing that it is safer, wanting to avoid unnecessary medical interventions, previous negative hospital experiences, wanting more control over the birthing experience, wanting to be in a comfortable and familiar environment, and having trust in the body's natural birthing process.[53] These desires are understandable, and everyone should have the right to choose where they feel safest giving birth. However, it is important to emphasize that home births – especially unattended home births, which make up one-fourth (25%) of home births in the United States – carry risks.[54] Planned home births have been linked to increased rates of health problems/complications and death among babies. These include risks such as neonatal seizures, serious neurological problems, and low Agpar scores.[54,55] These increased risks are in part due to lack of timely access to necessary medical interventions if childbirth complications arise – which can happen very quickly, even in previously uncomplicated pregnancies. The American College of Obstetricians and Gynecologists advises that there are certain higher risk groups who should never attempt a planned home birth, including those with past histories of C-section, those carrying multiple babies, and those whose babies are not positioned for a head-first delivery.[54] Research has also suggested that the risk of negative outcomes is higher among those who are giving birth for the first time, and in late- and post-term pregnancies (41 weeks gestation and beyond).[54,55]

Take Action

Imagine that your pregnant client expresses a desire to have a home birth. How might you respond in a way that is respectful, compassionate, and informative?

Freestanding community birth centers are another option for out-of-hospital births. In the United States, community birth centers are often run by midwives and emphasize holistic care and low-intervention childbirth. Evidence regarding outcomes in these settings is mixed. For example, a large study in the United States found that giving birth at a birthing center (rather than a hospital) was related to a significantly higher rates of infant health complications and death.[55] Alternatively, other research has suggested that, for those living in rural areas with relatively low-risk pregnancies, midwife-led community birth is not associated with increased health risks.[56] Another multi-year study of Medicaid (public insurance) recipients across the United States found that those who gave birth at community birth centers actually had lower rates of C-section, preterm birth, and low birthweight than those with similar profiles who gave birth in other settings.[57] A notable example, the Roots Community Birth Center in urban Minnesota, is designed to provide culturally centered, individualized, high-quality care for people of color, especially Black women. Roots accepts Medicaid (insurance) and employs certified nurse midwives and certified professional midwives who provide prenatal care, childbirth support, and general physical and reproductive healthcare.[58] Full-spectrum doula support is also available. Remarkably, as of 2020 when Roots had been operating for four years, the center had a 0% preterm birth rate.[59]

Taken together, these findings suggest that, while birthing centers may be a viable option for those with relatively low risk factors, it is very important to carefully weigh the potential risks, benefits, and quality of potential birthing facilities.

Healthcare During the Postpartum Period

Tatiana's Story ♥

Tatiana, a 37-year-old first-time mother, arrived at her six-week postpartum check-up looking forward to talking to her obstetrician/gynecologist, Dr. Green. Tatiana had a fairly uncomplicated vaginal delivery, though she did require stitching for a second-degree tear. The place where she tore was still swollen and uncomfortable, and she was nervous about resuming intimacy with her partner. In the last few weeks, she had also been feeling more anxious than usual and having trouble quieting her mind, especially before bedtime.

When the exam room door opened, Tatiana was surprised to see someone other than Dr. Green. "I'm Dr. Matthews, one of Dr. Green's students," he said. "Since everything went smoothly with the birth, we thought I'd go ahead and do this appointment if that's OK with you." Before Tatiana could respond, he motioned for her to slide down to the end of the exam table. He quickly examined her and said, "Stitches look good and you're healing well. Any questions?"

"Well, it's still pretty sore down there . . . " Tatiana began.

"That's to be expected. It can take some time for things to get back to normal." Dr. Matthews interrupted. "But if you notice any signs of infection, give us a call." He proceeded to ask a few basic questions about other topics. "And how is your mood? Any feelings of depression or hopelessness?"

"No," Tatiana said. "But I do feel more worked up than usual. I've got a million things running through my mind and I worry I'm going to forget something . . . ."

"Sounds like you're a new mom," Dr. Matthews said. "It's normal to feel stressed. Make sure you're getting enough sleep and getting outside – the fresh air will be good for you and baby. Otherwise – sounds like everything's going well. I'll refill your prescription for the birth control pill and you'll be on your way."

Key Term

The "fourth trimester": The 12-week period after giving birth.

According to Columbia University's Irving Medical Center,

> The fourth trimester – the 12 weeks after giving birth – is just as important for a mother's health as the first three trimesters. Yet this is often when mothers have the least interaction with their healthcare team, a time when, some experts argue, mothers need it the most.[60]

Indeed, during the fourth trimester, parents are adjusting to their new identity, whether they are new parents or have added a child to their family. They are getting to know and understand the new baby and help their family adjust to new routines, all the while continuing to experience physical and cognitive changes – particularly if they have given birth. This is a vital time when community and social service providers can make a difference in helping clients access the care and support they and their families need.

The American College of Obstetricians and Gynecologists recommends that several healthcare appointments occur in the "fourth trimester," depending on one's individual situation and needs.[61] Importantly, this includes those who have experienced miscarriage, stillbirth, or neonatal death. In most cases, the first check-in should occur about three weeks after giving birth, and a more comprehensive exam should occur no later than 12 weeks postpartum. During this examination, a healthcare provider should assess the physical, psychological, and social well-being of the postpartum patient.[61] Ideally, they will also provide individualized counseling around any pregnancy- or childbirth-related health problems or complications (i.e., gestational diabetes, injuries sustained during childbirth), as well as any chronic medical conditions (i.e., obesity, Type 1 or Type 2 diabetes, SUD). They may also make referrals to specialized support services, such as pelvic floor physical therapy, mental healthcare, lactation support, or food assistance.

Unfortunately, as highlighted by Tatiana's story, many feel rushed or unheard during their postpartum healthcare appointments. These appointments are often quite brief, and as a result, providers may prioritize some topics more than others.[62] For example, research has found that while postpartum depression screenings are often highly prioritized, screenings for intimate partner violence and substance use are less commonly conducted.[63] In other studies, postpartum patients reported that they wished their healthcare providers spent more time on topics related to mental health, sexual health, and adjusting to parenthood.[64,65]

Meanwhile, parents whose newborns are in the NICU often present with particular health concerns (i.e., colds, coughs, migraines, mental health needs) that need to be addressed during postpartum visits.[66] Whenever possible, maintaining continuous care with the same healthcare provider from pregnancy through the postpartum period can help ensure seamless care and attention to each patient's unique needs.[67,68]

Specialized Postpartum Care

Postpartum healthcare needs can look different based on several factors, such as how complicated the delivery was, pre-existing health conditions, and more. For example, in the United States, many patients who give birth in a hospital are discharged within three days unless they have severe complications – even if they underwent a C-section. Research has found that those who have had C-sections are at increased risk for complications, and that a small but substantial percentage need to visit the emergency room or even be readmitted to the hospital in the weeks after giving birth.[69,70]

Another noteworthy group that requires specialized postpartum care is those with HIV. This group is at increased risk for postpartum health complications such as infection, sepsis, and need for blood transfusions.[71] They also commonly face stigma in both their everyday lives and in healthcare settings, and as such may benefit from additional social and mental health supports during the postpartum period.[72] Research has found that women living with HIV are at increased risk for falling out of touch with the healthcare system after giving birth, and for viral rebound.[73,74] Individualized case management has been found to be helpful for keeping individuals with HIV engaged in the healthcare system during the postpartum period.[75] Similar approaches can be applied to those with other risk factors during pregnancy and the postpartum period, such as individuals with a history of substance use.

Take Time to Reflect

Consider how you could support clients in bringing questions and concerns to their postpartum healthcare appointments. For example, many people find it helpful to write down their questions and concerns in advance, so that they can easily refer to their notes if they forget what they wanted to say or become flustered.

Disparities in Postpartum Care Access

Despite the importance of postpartum healthcare, many struggle to attend these appointments for a variety of reasons. These reasons are often influenced by SDOH, like access to transportation, insurance, and time off from employment. Studies have suggested that anywhere between one-third and one-half of individuals do not attend any postpartum visits, and that every missed appointment increases the risk of future missed appointments.[76,77,78,79] Non-attendance rates have been found to be higher among patients with Medicaid (public insurance) or no insurance, those who were Hispanic/Latinx, those who had vaginal deliveries, and adolescents.[78] Loss of insurance coverage has also been found to be a significant barrier to postpartum care access.[80]

Similarly, researchers in a different study found that women who were younger, single, had lower levels of education, had lower socioeconomic resources, did not have insurance, and/or who smoked were least likely to receive postpartum care. Women who gave birth out of hospital and those who received inadequate prenatal care were also less likely to receive postpartum care.[81] A separate study found several other strong predictors of non-attendance, such as experiencing infant loss, not receiving dental care, and working during pregnancy.[82] Other research has similarly found that women of color are less likely to complete the transition from obstetric (pregnancy-related) care to primary care during the postpartum period, which may increase the risk of health problems/complications.[83] This trend is almost certainly related to SDOH and experiences with medical bias and racism. For example, one national study in the United States found that women who had experienced discrimination in the healthcare system due to their race or ethnicity, insurance type, or a difference of opinion with their provider were more than twice as likely to not attend postpartum visits.[84]

Numerous interventions to increase postpartum visit attendance have been investigated. For example, one study reported on the findings of a postpartum navigation program at a clinic that primarily served patients of color with Medicaid (public insurance). The clinic employed a "navigator" whose job was to provide support and logistical assistance to postpartum patients. Findings linked this program to significantly higher rates of postpartum visit attendance, as well as increased rates of depression screening, vaccinations, and contraceptive use.[85] Another intervention, Strong Start for Mothers and Newborns, used many strategies to promote continuous care from pregnancy through the postpartum period such as addressing information gaps, linking patients to resources, addressing transportation and childcare needs, and providing incentives for postpartum care. Research suggested that this program increased access to postpartum care among people with Medicaid (public insurance).[86] Telehealth appointments have also found promise for appointments that do not require a physical examination, and text-messaging reminders have also been found to be helpful.[87,88,89,90] Taken together, these findings suggest that interventions that address SDOH can play a significant role in improving postpartum care access.

Putting It Into Practice

- ***Discuss stressors and the range of emotions that come with having a new baby – before and after baby is born.*** As a community or social service provider, you can provide families with a safe space to discuss the stressors and range of feelings that a new baby brings – for example, the very real impacts of sleep deprivation, and healing from a major medical event. By discussing these topics early and often, you can encourage open communication and normalize parents' experiences, while also keeping an eye out for signs that someone may be experiencing something more significant, such as postpartum depression or anxiety. Because you likely work with families for an extended period and with some frequency, you are well-situated to help identify mental health challenges in the fourth trimester and beyond.

- ***As the due date approaches, plan how you will check in with families after the birth.*** Explore the family's preferences – do they think they would like to see you in person soon after birth, or to check in virtually and wait to meet in person for a couple of weeks? Let them know that it is common for preferences to change after giving birth – you are flexible and available.
- ***If the family is agreeable, check in with them in person or virtually following delivery.*** The first days at home following a birth can be emotional and stressful, on top of the experience of physically recovering from giving birth. During these early days, families may be especially receptive to assistance from those with whom they already have established trusting relationships. During this time, offer emotional support and connections to critical resources like lactation consultation. Encourage parents to follow-up with healthcare providers about any health concerns or symptoms for themselves or their newborn.
- ***Share information about physical and emotional changes during the postpartum period.*** When you are equipped with an understanding of typical physical and emotional changes, as well as red flags in the postpartum period (Table 7.1), you can help families better understand their postpartum experiences. You can also help identify when a family's experience is of concern and warrants additional attention or intervention.

Table 7.1 Changes That Can Occur After Giving Birth

Physical changes that can occur after giving birth[91]	*Emotional changes that can occur after giving birth*[92]
• Vaginal discharge • Contractions or cramping • Trouble or pain during urination • Vaginal soreness • Night sweats • Engorgement and sore breasts • Skin, hair and weight changes • Fatigue	• Increased stress • The baby blues • Typical adjustment reaction (an extension of the baby blues through the first two months after birth) • Postpartum exhaustion • Postpartum depression and/or anxiety *Reminder:* postpartum mental health is discussed in detail in Chapter 3.

- ***Support postpartum mental health.*** Major health organizations advise that healthcare providers should screen everyone for depression symptoms at their postpartum check-up. However, this timepoint may miss those who do not attend a postpartum check-up, those who experience depression symptoms later in the postpartum period, or those who are experiencing anxiety or other types of mental health challenges. Home visits and other touchpoints with community and social service providers can be ideal opportunities to conduct mental health screenings and make referrals if needed. As mentioned throughout this book, community and social service providers can begin by providing all clients with education about mental health in the postpartum period, and then conduct screenings with clients and co-parents/partners who may also be experiencing postpartum mental health challenges. Major transitions like going back to work, sleep regressions, or weaning from breastfeeding may be particularly poignant times to check in.

- ***Encourage pregnant and postpartum clients to lean on their social support systems.*** Retaining a sense of community with family members, friends, neighbors, and others can be very helpful during postpartum adjustment. As mentioned in Chapter 3, there is some evidence that those whose levels of social support go down during the postpartum period are at increased risk for depression, whereas those who stay connected to their support systems are more likely to maintain good mental health. The same study found that joining new social groups during the postpartum period did not make a significant difference in the risk of depression. With the pressures and demands that come with caring for a newborn, it is easy to understand how challenging it can be for parents to stay connected socially. However, by talking with families about how important these social supports are for mental health and well-being, parents may be more motivated.
- ***Make connections to specialized support services.*** You can raise awareness of other support services – for example, pelvic floor physical therapy, lactation support, and more. In some cases, the parent may need to ask their healthcare provider for a referral; in others, you may be able to provide a direct referral or warm hand-off.

Doula Care

One promising strategy for improving experiences during childbirth and the postpartum period is doula care. A doula is a non-medical professional who has been trained to provide support, education, and advocacy during pregnancy, childbirth, and/or the postpartum period. A full-spectrum doula provides these services from pregnancy through postpartum.[93] Doulas can help clients advocate for themselves and can also advocate on their behalf as requested. During childbirth, doulas can help communicate the client's birthing plan or wishes, be another set of eyes and ears, and offer support and comfort.

Research has linked doula care to better maternal and infant outcomes, such as more respectful care from healthcare providers, lower rates of preterm birth and C-sections, shorter labors, and lower levels of stress and anxiety.[94,95,96,97] Doula care can be especially valuable for people of color, particularly if they are matched with a doula from a similar background who understands the disparities and discrimination present in healthcare settings.[98,99,100,101,102,103,104] Other populations with unique health needs – such as adolescents, those who identify as LGBTQ+, and those struggling with substance use – have also been found to benefit from doula support.[105,106] While working with a doula has often been inaccessible due to cost, states are increasingly covering doula services through Medicaid.[107]

Putting It Into Practice

- ***Integrate doula services.*** Community and social service organizations can increase access to doula services by incorporating doulas into the continuum of services they offer. Some community and social service providers choose to become trained as doulas and offer these services to clients directly. Some organizations hire doulas as staff, while others partner with individual doulas or doula agencies to offer these services to client families as needed. These are just a few examples of how doula services can be integrated within community and social services to improve health outcomes.

Your Role as a Community or Social Service Provider

Listening and Learning

The data and information in this chapter present a picture of key issues related to health and healthcare during childbirth and the year after giving birth. Understanding the data, statistics, and stories specific to your community will help you tailor your services to the issues, needs, and strengths of your local community and the families within it. Consider: what do you already know about the healthcare experiences of people in your community during childbirth and postpartum (for example, availability of doula services, rates of childbirth interventions such as unplanned C-sections, out-of-hospital births)? How can you learn more (i.e., researching information and local data, listening to personal stories of different kinds of families in your community, etc.)?

Advocating

As discussed earlier in this book, your role as a community or service provider operates on two levels: (a) your individual work with families; and (b) your work with systems, including local healthcare providers, clinics, and networks. The lessons outlined here pertain to both levels of work and point to the need for advocacy to reduce medical bias and expand the continuum of quality healthcare options available during childbirth and the postpartum period. You can be an advocate within your organization – for example, by proactively identifying culturally responsive healthcare providers, by engaging in professional development about recognizing and addressing medical bias, or by encouraging your organization to integrate additional services, such as doulas.

You can also advocate outside of your organization in the community at large by lifting up policies, programs, and initiatives designed to combat bias in the medical system and improve childbirth and postpartum safety and success.

Take Time to Reflect

Reflecting on the practice implications throughout this chapter and your role as a community or social service provider, what is one area where you believe you are already doing an excellent job? What is one area where you could improve your professional practice or deepen your knowledge and understanding?

Take Action

Now that you have reflected on an area where you could improve your professional practice, create a SMART goal to make it happen. Remember, a SMART goal is described as follows.

- **S**pecific
- **M**easurable
- **A**chievable
- **R**elevant
- **T**ime-Bound

For example, imagine that you have noticed that many of your clients do not attend their postpartum check-ups. A SMART goal might be:

> Many of my clients do not attend their postpartum check-ups because they forget, or they do not have transportation or childcare. I know that attending these check-ups is very important for their recovery (**Relevant**). This month (**Time-Bound**), I will check in with all four of my newly postpartum clients and make sure they have a postpartum check-up scheduled. I'll encourage them to put a calendar reminder on their phone and ask if they need any help with transportation or childcare (**Specific, Achievable**). My goal is that at least three of them (75%) will make it to their check-up (**Measurable**).

Key Takeaways From This Chapter

1. Many individuals feel unsupported, unheard, and even mistreated by the healthcare and birthing professionals who are supposed to take care of them during childbirth. These experiences are often related to bias in healthcare systems, and among individual healthcare providers.
2. Elective labor induction, elective C-section, and out-of-hospital births all carry health risks. Individuals who are considering these procedures or receiving recommendations for them should carefully discuss the potential risks and benefits, and their unique situations, with their healthcare provider.
3. Postpartum healthcare is an important part of the physical and mental recovery process; however, many do not attend these visits because of negative healthcare experiences, transportation or childcare challenges, or other reasons outside of their individual control. Community and social service providers can play an important role in encouraging their postpartum clients to follow-up with their healthcare providers and how to navigate barriers that may exist to accessing care.

References

1. Dwyer, D., & See, P. (2023, November). *'Nobody cared': Women who have reported mistreatment while giving birth say CDC report validates their trauma*. ABC News. https://abcnews.go.com/Politics/cared-women-reported-mistreatment-giving-birth-cdc-report/story?id=105077279

2. Greenfield, B. (2017, March). *Woman forced into violent episiotomy settles with doctor*. Yahoo. www.yahoo.com/lifestyle/woman-forced-into-violent-episiotomy-settles-with-doctor-182947205.html
3. Hartney, M. (n.d.). *Kimberly said no*. www.michellehartney.com/kimberly-said-no
4. Demirel, G., Kaya, N., & Evcili, F. (2022). The relationship between women's perception of support and control during childbirth on fear of birth and mother's satisfaction. *Journal of Obstetrics and Gynaecology*, *42*(1), 83–90. https://doi.org/10.1080/01443615.2021.1882970
5. Lunda, P., Minnie, C. S., & Benadé, P. (2018). Women's experiences of continuous support during childbirth: a meta-synthesis. *BMC Pregnancy and Childbirth*, *18*(1), 1–11. https://doi.org/10.1186/s12884-018-1755-8
6. Simon, R. M., Johnson, K. M., & Liddell, J. (2016). Amount, source, and quality of support as predictors of women's birth evaluations. *Birth*, *43*(3), 226–232. https://doi.org/10.1111/birt.12227
7. DeBaets, A. M. (2017). From birth plan to birth partnership: enhancing communication in childbirth. *American Journal of Obstetrics and Gynecology*, *216*(1), 31.e1–31.e4. https://doi.org/10.1016/j.ajog.2016.09.087
8. Wang, E., Glazer, K. B., Sofaer, S., Balbierz, A., & Howell, E. A. (2021). Racial and ethnic disparities in severe maternal morbidity: A qualitative study of women's experiences of peripartum care. *Women's Health Issues*, *31*(1), 75–81. https://doi.org/10.1016/j.whi.2020.09.002
9. Hemphill, N. O., Crooks, N., Zhang, W., Fitter, F., Erbe, K., Rutherford, J. N., Liese, K. L., Pearson, P., Stewart, K., Kessee, N., Reed, L., Tussing-Humphreys, L., & Koenig, M. D. (2023). Obstetric experiences of young black mothers: An intersectional perspective. *Social Science & Medicine (1982)*, *317*, 115604. https://doi.org/10.1016/j.socscimed.2022.115604
10. Roder-DeWan, S., Baril, N., Belanoff, C. M., Declercq, E. R., & Langer, A. (2021). Being known: A grounded theory study of the meaning of quality maternity care to people of color in Boston. *Journal of Midwifery & Women's Health*, *66*(4), 452–458. https://doi.org/10.1111/jmwh.13240
11. Louis, M. S., Mangal, R. K., Stead, T. S., Jones, T., & Ganti, L. (2023). Racial disparities in satisfaction with maternal healthcare. *Journal of the National Medical Association*, *115*(6), 589–592. https://doi.org/10.1016/j.jnma.2023.10.001
12. Attanasio, L. B., Kozhimannil, K. B., & Kjerulff, K. H. (2018). Factors influencing women's perceptions of shared decision making during labor and delivery: Results from a large-scale cohort study of first childbirth. *Patient Education and Counseling*, *101*(6), 1130–1136. https://doi.org/10.1016/j.pec.2018.01.002
13. Logan, R. G., McLemore, M. R., Julian, Z., Stoll, K., Malhotra, N., GVtM Steering Council, & Vedam, S. (2022). Coercion and non-consent during birth and newborn care in the United States. *Birth*, *49*(4), 749–762. https://doi.org/10.1111/birt.12641
14. Altman, M. R., McLemore, M. R., Oseguera, T., Lyndon, A., & Franck, L. S. (2020). Listening to women: Recommendations from women of color to improve experiences in pregnancy and birth care. *Journal of Midwifery & Women's Health*, *65*(4), 466–473. https://doi.org/10.1111/jmwh.13102
15. Lothian, J. A. (2019). Safe childbirth: A call to action. *The Journal of Perinatal Education*, *28*(2), 65–67. https://doi.org/10.1891/1058-1243.28.2.65
16. West, R., & Barkowski, J. P. (2019). Negotiating patient-provider power dynamics in distinct childbirth settings: Insights from Black American mothers. *Societies*, *9*(2), 45. https://doi.org/10.3390/soc9020045
17. Kalata, M., Kalata, K., Yen, H., Khorshid, A., Davis, T., & Meredith, J. (2020). Community perspectives on the racial disparity in perinatal outcomes. *The Journal of Maternal-Fetal & Neonatal Medicine*, 1–6. https://doi.org/10.1080/14767058.2020.1786525
18. Molina, R. L., Beecroft, A., Pazos Herencia, Y., Bazan, M., Wade, C., DiMeo, A., Sprankle, J., & Sullivan, M. M. (2024). Pregnancy care utilization, experiences, and outcomes among undocumented immigrants in the United States: A scoping review. *Women's Health Issues*, *34*(4), 370–380. https://doi.org/10.1016/j.whi.2024.02.001
19. Griggs, K. M., Waddill, C. B., Bice, A., & Ward, N. (2021). Care during pregnancy, childbirth, postpartum, and human milk feeding for individuals who identify as LGBTQ. *MCN. The American Journal of Maternal Child Nursing*, *46*(1), 43–53. https://doi.org/10.1097/NMC.0000000000000675

20. Heggie, C., Cowal, G., MacIntosh, C., & Paynter, M. (2023). Supportive and affirming queer perinatal health care: A qualitative study. *LGBTQ+ Family: An Interdisciplinary Journal, 19*(5), 405–415. https://doi.org/10.1080/27703371.2023.2242319
21. Roosevelt, L. K., Pietzmeier, S., & Reed, R. (2021). Clinically and culturally competent care for transgender and nonbinary people: A challenge to providers of perinatal care. *The Journal of Perinatal & Neonatal Nursing, 35*(2), 142–149. https://doi.org/10.1097/JPN.0000000000000560
22. Malmquist, A., Jonsson, L., Wikström, J., & Nieminen, K. (2019). Minority stress adds an additional layer to fear of childbirth in lesbian and bisexual women, and transgender people. *Midwifery, 79*, 102551. https://doi.org/10.1016/j.midw.2019.102551
23. Wheeler, V., Hoffman, A., & Bybel, M. (2022). Cervical ripening and induction of labor. *American Family Physician, 105*(2), 177–186.
24. Mayo Clinic (2024). *Labor and delivery, postpartum care*. www.mayoclinic.org/healthy-lifestyle/labor-and-delivery/in-depth/inducing-labor/art-20047557
25. Teitler, J. O., Plaza, R., Hegyi, T., Kruse, L., & Reichman, N. E. (2019). Elective deliveries and neonatal outcomes in full-term pregnancies. *American Journal of Epidemiology, 188*(4), 674–683. https://doi.org/10.1093/aje/kwz014
26. Langen, E. S., Schiller, A. J., Moore, K., Jiang, C., Bourdeau, A., Morgan, D. M., & Low, L. K. (2024). Outcomes of elective induction of labor at 39 weeks from a statewide collaborative quality initiative. *American Journal of Perinatology, 41*(S01), e1281–e1287. https://doi.org/10.1055/s-0043-1761918
27. Little, S. E. (2017). Elective induction of labor: What is the impact? *Obstetrics and Gynecology Clinics of North America, 44*(4), 601–614. https://doi.org/10.1016/j.ogc.2017.08.005
28. American College of Obstetricians and Gynecologists and the Society for Maternal-Fetal Medicine, Caughey, A. B., Cahill, A. G., Guise, J., & Rouse, D. J. (2014). Safe prevention of the primary cesarean delivery. *American Journal of Obstetricians & Gynecology, 210*(3), 179–193. https://doi.org/10.1016/j.ajog.2014.01.026
29. The American College of Obstetricians and Gynecologists (2013, April). *Cesarean delivery on maternal request*. www.acog.org/clinical/clinical-guidance/committee-opinion/articles/2019/01/cesarean-delivery-on-maternal-request
30. Lavecchia, M., Sabbah, M., & Abenhaim, H. A. (2016). Effect of planned mode of delivery in women with advanced maternal age. *Maternal and Child Health Journal, 20*(11), 2318–2327. https://doi.org/10.1007/s10995-016-2055-4
31. Kamath, B. D., Todd, J. K., Glazner, J. E., Lezotte, D., & Lynch, A. M. (2009). Neonatal outcomes after elective cesarean delivery. *Obstetrics and Gynecology, 113*(6), 1231–1238. https://doi.org/10.1097/AOG.0b013e3181a66d57
32. Rikhardsdottir, J. V., Hardardottir, H., & Thorkelsson, T. (2021). The majority of early term elective cesarean sections can be postponed. *The Journal of Maternal-Fetal & Neonatal Medicine, 34*(20), 3344–3349. https://doi.org/10.1080/14767058.2019.1684467
33. Liu, S., Liston, R. M., Joseph, K. S., Heaman, M., Sauve, R., Kramer, M. S., & Maternal Health Study Group of the Canadian Perinatal Surveillance System (2007). Maternal mortality and severe morbidity associated with low-risk planned cesarean delivery versus planned vaginal delivery at term. *Canadian Medical Association Journal, 176*(4), 455–460. https://doi.org/10.1503/cmaj.060870
34. The American College of Obstetricians and Gynecologists. *Cesarean birth*. www.acog.org/womens-health/faqs/cesarean-birth#:~:text=Cesarean%20birth%20also%20increases%20risks,the%20surgery%20outweigh%20the%20risks
35. Fresch, R., Stephens, K., & DeFranco, E. (2024). The combined influence of maternal medical conditions on the risk of primary cesarean delivery. *AJP Reports, 14*(1), e51–e56. https://doi.org/10.1055/s-0043-1777996
36. Richards, M. K., Flanagan, M. R., Littman, A. J., Burke, A. K., & Callegari, L. S. (2016). Primary cesarean section and adverse delivery outcomes among women of very advanced maternal age. *Journal of Perinatology, 36*(4), 272–277. https://doi.org/10.1038/jp.2015.204
37. Witt, W. P., Wisk, L. E., Cheng, E. R., Mandell, K., Chatterjee, D., Wakeel, F., Godecker, A. L., & Zarak, D. (2015). Determinants of cesarean delivery in the US: A lifecourse approach. *Maternal and Child Health Journal, 19*(1), 84–93. https://doi.org/10.1007/s10995-014-1498-8

38. Vanderlaan, J., Edwards, J. A., & Dunlop, A. (2020). Geospatial variation in caesarean delivery. *Nursing Open*, *7*(2), 627–633. https://doi.org/10.1002/nop2.433
39. Teal, E. N., Baer, R. J., Jelliffe-Pawlowski, L., & Mengesha, B. (2024). Racial disparities in cesarean delivery rates: Do hospital-level factors matter? *American Journal of Perinatology*, *41*(4), 375–382. https://doi.org/10.1055/s-0043-1776346
40. Teal, E. N., Anudokem, K., Baer, R. J., Jelliffe-Pawlowski, L., & Mengesha, B. (2024). Racial disparities in the rates of and indications for cesarean delivery in California: Are they changing over time? *American Journal of Perinatology*, *41*(1), 31–38. https://doi.org/10.1055/s-0041-1740071
41. Clark, R. R. S., Peele, M. E., Srinivas, S., & Lake, E. T. (2024). Racial disparities in low-risk cesarean birth rates across hospitals. *Birth*, *51*(1), 176–185. https://doi.org/10.1111/birt.12778
42. Hanson, C., Samson, K., Anderson-Berry, A. L., Slotkowski, R. A., & Su, D. (2022). Racial disparities in caesarean delivery among nulliparous women that delivered at term: Cross-sectional decomposition analysis of Nebraska birth records from 2005–2014. *BMC Pregnancy and Childbirth*, *22*(1), 329. https://doi.org/10.1186/s12884-022-04666-3
43. Williams, A., Little, S. E., Bryant, A. S., & Smith, N. A. (2024). Mode of delivery and unplanned cesarean: Differences in rates and indication by race, ethnicity, and sociodemographic characteristics. *American Journal of Perinatology*, *41*(7), 834–841. https://doi.org/10.1055/a-1785-8843
44. Stark, E. L., Grobman, W. A., & Miller, E. S. (2021). The association between maternal race and ethnicity and risk factors for primary cesarean delivery in nulliparous women. *American Journal of Perinatology*, *38*(4), 350–356. https://doi.org/10.1055/s-0039-1697587
45. Tangel, V., White, R. S., Nachamie, A. S., & Pick, J. S. (2019). Racial and ethnic disparities in maternal outcomes and the disadvantage of peripartum black women: A multistate analysis, 2007–2014. *American Journal of Perinatology*, *36*(8), 835–848. https://doi.org/10.1055/s-0038-1675207
46. Glazer, K. B., Danilack, V. A., Werner, E. F., Field, A. E., & Savitz, D. A. (2020). Elucidating the role of overweight and obesity in racial and ethnic disparities in cesarean delivery risk. *Annals of Epidemiology*, *42*, 4–11. https://doi.org/10.1016/j.annepidem.2019.12.012
47. Neal, J. L., Carlson, N. S., Phillippi, J. C., Tilden, E. L., Smith, D. C., Breman, R. B., Dietrich, M.S., & Lowe, N. K. (2019). Midwifery presence in United States medical centers and labor care and birth outcomes among low-risk nulliparous women: A consortium on safe labor study. *Birth*, *46*(3), 475–486. https://doi.org/10.1111/birt.12407
48. Smith, D. C., Phillippi, J. C., Lowe, N. K., Breman, R. B., Carlson, N. S., Neal, J. L., Gutierrez, E., & Tilden, E. L. (2020). Using the Robson 10-group classification system to compare cesarean birth utilization between US centers with and without midwives. *Journal of Midwifery & Women's Health*, *65*(1), 10–21. https://doi.org/10.1111/jmwh.13035
49. The American College of Obstetricians and Gynecologists (2019, February). *Approaches to limit intervention during labor and birth.* www.acog.org/clinical/clinical-guidance/committee-opinion/articles/2019/02/approaches-to-limit-intervention-during-labor-and-birth
50. Phillips, S. E. K., Celi, A. C., Wehbe, A., Kaduthodil, J., & Zera, C. A. (2023). Mobilizing the fourth trimester to improve population health: Interventions for postpartum transitions of care. *American Journal of Obstetrics and Gynecology*, *229*(1), 33–38. https://doi.org/10.1016/j.ajog.2022.12.309
51. MacDorman, M. F., & Declercq, E. (2019). Trends and state variations in out-of-hospital births in the United States, 2004–2017. *Birth*, *46*(2), 279–288. https://doi.org/10.1111/birt.12411v
52. Kozhimannil, K. B., Hung, P., Henning-Smith, C., Casey, M. M., & Prasad, S. (2018). Association between loss of hospital-based obstetric services and birth outcomes in rural counties in the United States. *JAMA*, *319*(12), 1239–1247. https://doi.org/10.1001/jama.2018.1830
53. Descieux, K., Kavasseri, K., Scott, K., & Parlier, A. B. (2017). Why women choose home birth: A narrative review. *MAHEC Online Journal of Research*, *3*(2).
54. The American College of Obstetricians and Gynecologists (2017, April). *Planned home birth.* www.acog.org/clinical/clinical-guidance/committee-opinion/articles/2017/04/planned-home-birth

55. Grünebaum, A., McCullough, L. B., Sapra, K. J., Brent, R. L., Levene, M. I., Arabin, B., & Chervenak, F. A. (2013). Apgar score of 0 at 5 minutes and neonatal seizures or serious neurologic dysfunction in relation to birth setting. *American Journal of Obstetrics and Gynecology, 209*(4), 323.e1–323.e3236. https://doi.org/10.1016/j.ajog.2013.06.025
56. Nethery, E., Gordon, W., Bovbjerg, M. L., & Cheyney, M. (2018). Rural community birth: maternal and neonatal outcomes for planned community births among rural women in the United States, 2004–2009. *Birth, 45*(2), 120–129. https://doi.org/10.1111/birt.12322
57. Alliman, J., Stapleton, S. R., Wright, J., Bauer, K., Slider, K., & Jolles, D. (2019). Strong Start in birth centers: Socio-demographic characteristics, care processes, and outcomes for mothers and newborns. *Birth, 46*(2), 234–243. https://doi.org/10.1111/birt.12433
58. Almanza, J. I., Karbeah, J., Tessier, K. M., Neerland, C., Stoll, K., Hardeman, R. R., & Vedam, S. (2022). The impact of culturally-centered care on peripartum experiences of autonomy and respect in community birth centers: A comparative study. *Maternal and Child Health Journal, 26*(4), 895–904. https://doi.org/10.1007/s10995-021-03245-w
59. Hardeman, R. R., Almanza, J., & Kozhimannil, K. B. (2020). Roots community birth center: A culturally-centered care model for improving value and equity in childbirth. *Healthcare, 8*(1), 100367. https://doi.org/10.1016/j.hjdsi.2019.100367
60. Columbia University Irving Medical Center (2021, November). *A mother's guide to the fourth trimester.* www.cuimc.columbia.edu/news/mothers-guide-fourth-trimester#:~:text=The%20fourth%20trimester%%20E2%80%94the%2012,mothers%20need%20it%20the%20most
61. The American College of Obstetricians and Gynecologists (2018). *Optimizing postpartum care.* www.acog.org/clinical/clinical-guidance/committee-opinion/articles/2018/05/optimizing-postpartum-care
62. Tully, K. P., Stuebe, A. M., & Verbiest, S. B. (2017). The fourth trimester: A critical transition period with unmet maternal health needs. *American Journal of Obstetrics and Gynecology, 217*(1), 37–41. https://doi.org/10.1016/j.ajog.2017.03.032
63. Krishnamurti, T., Simhan, H. N., & Borrero, S. (2020). Competing demands in postpartum care: A national survey of US providers' priorities and practice. *BMC Health Services Research, 20*, 1–10. https://doi.org/10.1186/s12913-020-05144-2
64. Guerra-Reyes, L., Christie, V. M., Prabhakar, A., & Siek, K. A. (2017). Mind the gap: Assessing the disconnect between postpartum health information desired and health information received. *Women's Health Issues, 27*(2), 167–173. https://doi.org/10.1016/j.whi.2016.11.004
65. Walker, L. O., & Francine Nichols, R. N. (2015). The broken thread of health promotion and disease prevention for women during the postpartum period. *The Journal of Perinatal Education, 24*(2), 81. https://doi.org/10.1891/1058-1243.24.2.81
66. Verbiest, S., Bonzon, E., & Handler, A. (2016). Postpartum health and wellness: A call for quality woman-centered care. *Maternal and Child Health Journal, 20*(1), 1–7. https://doi.org/10.1007/s10995-016-2188-5
67. Cornell, A., McCoy, C., Stampfel, C., Bonzon, E., & Verbiest, S. (2016). Creating new strategies to enhance postpartum health and wellness. *Maternal and Child Health Journal, 20*(1), 39–42. https://doi.org/10.1007/s10995-016-2182-y
68. Verbiest, S., Tully, K., Simpson, M., & Stuebe, A. (2018). Elevating mothers' voices: recommendations for improved patient-centered postpartum. *Journal of Behavioral Medicine, 41*(5), 577–590. https://doi.org/10.1007/s10865-018-9961-4
69. Oben, A., Perez, W., Jauk, V. C., Boggess, K., Clark, E., Saade, G., Esplin, M. S., Longo, S., Cleary, K. L., Wapner, R., Blackwell, S. C., Owens, M. Y., Ambalavanan, N., Szychowski, J. M., & Tita, A. (2022). Timing of maternal discharge after cesarean delivery and risk of maternal readmission. *American Journal of Perinatology, 39*(10), 1042–1047. https://doi.org/10.1055/s-0042-1743248
70. Rodriguez, A. N., Patel, S., Macias, D., Morgan, J., Kraus, A., & Spong, C. Y. (2021). Timing of emergency postpartum hospital visits in the fourth trimester. *American Journal of Perinatology, 38*(4), 319–325. https://doi.org/10.1055/s-0040-1716842
71. Arab, K., Spence, A. R., Czuzoj-Shulman, N., & Abenhaim, H. A. (2017). Pregnancy outcomes in HIV-positive women: A retrospective cohort study. *Archives of Gynecology and Obstetrics, 295*(3), 599–606. https://doi.org/10.1007/s00404-016-4271-y
72. Buchberg, M. K., Fletcher, F. E., Vidrine, D. J., Levison, J., Peters, M. Y., Hardwicke, R., Yu, X., & Bell, T. K. (2015). A mixed-methods approach to understanding barriers to postpartum

retention in care among low-income, HIV-infected women. *AIDS Patient Care and STDs*, *29*(3), 126–132. https://doi.org/10.1089/apc.2014.0227
73. Adhikari, E. H., Yule, C. S., Roberts, S. W., Rogers, V. L., Sheffield, J. S., Kelly, M. A., McIntire, D. D., & Barnes, A. (2019). Factors associated with postpartum loss to follow-up and detectable viremia after delivery among pregnant women living with HIV. *AIDS Patient Care and STDs*, *33*(1), 14–20. https://doi.org/10.1089/apc.2018.0117
74. Chen, J. S., Pence, B. W., Rahangdale, L., Patterson, K. B., Farel, C. E., Durr, A. L., Antono, A. C., Zakharova, O., Eron, J. J., & Napravnik, S. (2019). Postpartum HIV care continuum outcomes in the Southeastern US. *AIDS*, *33*(4), 637. https://doi.org/10.1097/QAD.0000000000002094
75. Hickman, A. B., Backus, K. V., Burns, P., & Brock, J. B. (2020). Evaluation of a postpartum linkage and retention quality improvement initiative for women living with HIV in the Deep South. *Journal of Public Health*, 1–7. https://doi.org/10.1007/s10389-020-01355-3
76. Wouk, K., Kinlaw, A. C., Farahi, N., Pfeifer, H., Yeatts, B., Paw, M. K., & Robinson, W. R. (2022). Correlates of receiving guideline-concordant postpartum health services in the community health center setting. *Women's Health Reports*, *3*(1), 180–193. https://doi.org/10.1089/whr.2021.0084
77. Christner, L. P., Irani, S., McGowan, C., Dabaja, E., Dejong, C., & Attar, M. A. (2023). Previous missed visits and independent risk of loss to follow-up in the high-risk neonatal follow-up clinic. *Early Human Development*, *183*, 105813. https://doi.org/10.1016/j.earlhumdev.2023.105813
78. Wilcox, A., Levi, E. E., & Garrett, J. M. (2016). Predictors of non-attendance to the postpartum follow-up visit. *Maternal and Child Health Journal*, *20*(1), 22–27. https://doi.org/10.1007/s10995-016-2184-9
79. Aqua, J. K., Ford, N. D., Pollack, L. M., Lee, J. S., Kuklina, E. V., Hayes, D. K., Vaughan, A. S., & Coronado, F. (2023). Timing of outpatient postpartum care utilization among women with chronic hypertension and hypertensive disorders of pregnancy. *American Journal of Obstetrics & Gynecology MFM*, *5*(9), 101051. https://doi.org/10.1016/j.ajogmf.2023.101051
80. Gemkow, J. W., Liss, D. T., Yang, T. Y., Padilla, R., King, P. L., Pereyra, S., Cox-Batson, S., Tenfelde, S., & Masinter, L. (2022). Predicting postpartum transition to primary care in community health centers. *American Journal of Preventive Medicine*, *63*(5), 689–699. https://doi.org/10.1016/j.amepre.2022.05.010
81. Danilack, V. A., Brousseau, E. C., Paulo, B. A., Matteson, K. A., & Clark, M. A. (2019). Characteristics of women without a postpartum checkup among PRAMS participants, 2009–2011. *Maternal and Child Health Journal*, *23*(7), 903–909. https://doi.org/10.1007/s10995-018-02716-x
82. Morgan, I., Hughes, M. E., Belcher, H., & Holmes, L. (2018). Maternal sociodemographic characteristics, experiences and health behaviors associated with postpartum care utilization: Evidence from Maryland PRAMS dataset, 2012–2013. *Maternal and Child Health Journal*, *22*(4), 589–598. https://doi.org/10.1007/s10995-018-2428-y
83. Essien, U. R., Molina, R. L., & Lasser, K. E. (2019). Strengthening the postpartum transition of care to address racial disparities in maternal health. *Journal of the National Medical Association*, *111*(4), 349–351. https://doi.org/10.1016/j.jnma.2018.10.016
84. Attanasio, L., & Kozhimannil, K. B. (2017). Health care engagement and follow-up after perceived discrimination in maternity care. *Medical Care*, *55*(9), 830–833. https://doi.org/10.1097/MLR.0000000000000773
85. Yee, L. M., Martinez, N. G., Nguyen, A. T., Hajjar, N., Chen, M. J., & Simon, M. A. (2017). Using a patient navigator to improve postpartum care in an urban women's health clinic. *Obstetrics and Gynecology*, *129*(5), 925. https://doi.org/10.1097/AOG.0000000000001977
86. Rodin, D., Silow-Carroll, S., Cross-Barnet, C., Courtot, B., & Hill, I. (2019). Strategies to promote postpartum visit attendance among Medicaid participants. *Journal of Women's Health*, *28*(9), 1246–1253. https://doi.org/10.1089/jwh.2018.7568
87. Saad, M., Chan, S., Nguyen, L., Srivastava, S., & Appireddy, R. (2021). Patient perceptions of the benefits and barriers of virtual postnatal care: A qualitative study. *BMC Pregnancy and Childbirth*, *21*(1), 543. https://doi.org/10.1186/s12884-021-03999-9
88. Dixon-Shambley, K., & Gabbe, P. T. (2021). Using telehealth approaches to address social determinants of health and improve pregnancy and postpartum outcomes. *Clinical Obstetrics and Gynecology*, *64*(2), 333–344. https://doi.org/10.1097/GRF.0000000000000611

89. Arias, M. P., Wang, E., Leitner, K., Sannah, T., Keegan, M., Delferro, J., Iluore, C., Arimoro, F., Streaty, T., & Hamm, R. F. (2022). The impact on postpartum care by telehealth: A retrospective cohort study. *American Journal of Obstetrics & Gynecology MFM*, *4*(3), 100611. https://doi.org/10.1016/j.ajogmf.2022.100611
90. Gomez, H. B., & Hoffman, M. K. (2021). Text messaging as a means to engage patients in the postpartum period. *Clinical Obstetrics and Gynecology*, *64*(2), 366–374. https://doi.org/10.1097/GRF.0000000000000609
91. Parents as Teachers National Center (n.d.). Parent educator resource: Postpartum recovery. In *Parents as Teachers Foundational Curriculum* (pp. 1744–1751). Parents as Teachers National Center.
92. Parents as Teachers National Center (n.d.). Parent educator resource: Postpartum adjustment. In *Parents as Teachers Foundational Curriculum* (pp. 1882–1886). Parents as Teachers National Center.
93. National Partnership for Women & Families. *"Our communities hold the solutions": The importance of full-spectrum doulas to reproductive health and justice.* https://nationalpartnership.org/wp-content/uploads/2023/04/our-communities-hold-the-solutions.pdf
94. Bihn-Coss, G., & Egbert, N. (2023). Supporting in solidarity: An examination of social support, advocacy, and barriers among birthing doulas. *Communication Quarterly*, *71*(3), 243–267. https://doi.org/10.1080/01463373.2022.2164737
95. Mallick, L. M., Thoma, M. E., & Shenassa, E. D. (2022). The role of doulas in respectful care for communities of color and Medicaid recipients. *Birth*, *49*(4), 823–832. https://doi.org/10.1111/birt.12655
96. Arteaga, S., Hubbard, E., Arcara, J., Cuentos, A., Armstead, M., Jackson, A., Gomez, A. M., & Marshall, C. (2023). "They're gonna be there to advocate for me so I'm not by myself": A qualitative analysis of Black women's motivations for seeking and experiences with community doula care. *Women and Birth: Journal of the Australian College of Midwives*, *36*(3), 257–263. https://doi.org/10.1016/j.wombi.2022.08.007
97. Thomas, M. P., Ammann, G., Onyebeke, C., Gomez, T. K., Lobis, S., Li, W., & Huynh, M. (2023). Birth equity on the front lines: Impact of a community-based doula program in Brooklyn, NY. *Birth*, *50*(1), 138–150. https://doi.org/10.1111/birt.12701
98. Kett, P. M., van Eijk, M. S., Guenther, G. A., & Skillman, S. M. (2022). "This work that we're doing is bigger than ourselves": A qualitative study with community-based birth doulas in the United States. *Perspectives on Sexual and Reproductive Health*, *54*(3), 99–108. https://doi.org/10.1363/psrh.12203
99. Reed, R., Nguyen, A., Armstead, M., Cuentos, A., Mystic, M.-I., Arcara, J., Jackson, A. V., Marshall, C., & Gomez, A. M. (2023). "An extra layer of pressure to be my best self": Healthcare provider perspectives on how doulas foster accountability and bridge gaps in pregnancy-related care. *SSM–Qualitative Research in Health*, *3*. https://doi.org/10.1016/j.ssmqr.2023.100259
100. Van Eijk, M. S., Guenther, G. A., Kett, P. M., Jopson, A. D., Frogner, B. K., & Skillman, S. M. (2022). Addressing systemic racism in birth doula services to reduce health inequities in the United States. *Health Equity*, *6*(1), 98–105. https://doi.org/10.1089/heq.2021.0033
101. Herriott, A. L., Etling, S., & Hans, S. L. (2024). Community-based doulas' roles within the birth support system: Young Black mothers' perspectives. *Journal of Midwifery & Women's Health*, *69*(1), 33–40. https://doi.org/10.1111/jmwh.13570
102. Kathawa, C. A., Arora, K. S., Zielinski, R., & Low, L. K. (2022). Perspectives of doulas of color on their role in alleviating racial disparities in birth outcomes: A qualitative study. *Journal of Midwifery & Women's Health*, *67*(1), 31–38. https://doi.org/10.1111/jmwh.13305
103. Nehme, E. K., Wilson, K. J., McGowan, R., Schuessler, K. R., Morse, S. M., & Patel, D. A. (2024). Providing doula support to publicly insured women in central Texas: A financial cost-benefit analysis. *Birth*, *51*(1), 63–70. https://doi.org/10.1111/birt.12766
104. Thomas, K., Quist, S., Peprah, S., Riley, K., Mittal, P. C., & Nguyen, B. T. (2023). The experiences of Black community-based doulas as they mitigate systems of racism: A qualitative study. *Journal of Midwifery & Women's Health*, *68*(4), 466–472. https://doi.org/10.1111/jmwh.13493
105. Heggie, C., Cowal, G., MacIntosh, C., & Paynter, M. (2023). Supportive and affirming queer perinatal health care: A qualitative study. *LGBTQ+ Family: An Interdisciplinary Journal*, *19*(5), 405–415. https://doi.org/10.1080/27703371.2023.2242319

106. Haerizadeh-Yazdi, N., Huynh, M. P., Narva, A., Grasty, A., Lemon, M., Claxton, N., Gillespie, K., & Kallem, S. (2023). Philadelphia Department of Health doula support program: Early successes and challenges of a program serving birthing people affected by substance use disorder. *Maternal and Child Health Journal*, *27*(Suppl 1), 52–57. https://doi.org/10.1007/s10995-023-03803-4
107. Mosley, E. A., Lindsey, A., Turner, D., Shah, P., Sayyad, A., Mack, A., & Lindberg, K. (2023). "I want . . . to serve those communities . . . [but] my price tag is . . . not what they can afford": The community-engaged Georgia doula study. *Perspectives on Sexual and Reproductive Health*, *55*(3), 200–209. https://doi.org/10.1363/psrh.12241

8 Healthcare and Breastfeeding During the First Year of Life

Self-Care Moment

Take a moment to release some tension through progressive muscle relaxation. Hold your hands in your lap with your palms facing upward. Imagine that you are holding a lemon in each hand. Now "squeeze the lemons" as tightly as you can, for at least ten seconds. Next, slowly open your hands. Feel the tension leaving your hands as you stretch your fingers and wrists.

Timely, high-quality healthcare is essential to ensuring the healthy growth and development of newborns and infants in the first year of life. For families that are breastfeeding, lactation support can also be valuable for ensuring their babies' nutritional needs are met. This chapter focuses on topics related to healthcare, lactation support, and parent education in the first year of life that are important for community and social service providers to know about, including discussion of research on this topic, practice implications for your work, and reflections on your role. You will also hear the stories of Devonte, a parent trying to get his infant daughter to a well-child check-up; Pooja, a new mother struggling with breastfeeding; and two PAT home visiting program affiliates with unique strategies for supporting health, healthcare, and breastfeeding in the first year of life.

Research Summary

Healthcare in the First Year of Life

Devonte's Story ♥

Devonte, a single parent of a baby girl named Dalia, was doing the best he could to juggle parenthood, his job as a middle school teacher, and supporting his elderly mother. But it was difficult, and both time and money were tight. He had very few sick days left at work and his car had recently broken down. And, while Dalia was doing well overall, Devonte noticed that her eyes sometimes seemed unfocused or crossed.

DOI: 10.4324/9781003476474-8

Devonte carefully scheduled Dalia's six-month well-child visit for 4 p.m. on a Friday so that he would have time to leave work, pick her up at daycare, and catch the city bus to the pediatrician's office. As luck would have it, he got stuck at work later than expected, causing him to be late to daycare pickup and to miss the bus. He called the pediatrician's office to see about rescheduling the appointment. "Unfortunately, we book out very far in advance," the receptionist said. "Our next opening is in eight weeks at 11 a.m. Will that work for you?"

It is recommended that newborns and infants attend multiple "well-child" healthcare appointments during the first year of life.[1] These appointments are important for ensuring that baby is growing and developing normally, and for identifying any potential health or developmental issues as early as possible. They typically include a head-to-toe exam, as well as conversations and screenings with the parent/caregiver.

The American Academy of Pediatrics recommends the following well-child visit schedule for most newborns and infants.[1]

- **First week**: The first check-up should occur at 3–5 days old; and
- **One, two, four, six, nine, and 12 months**: Check-ups should occur at each of these ages.

It is important to note that this recommended schedule is for children who are following typical development and have no major medical needs. Children with complex medical needs may need to be seen more often than this.

As with other recommended schedules of care, many families and children are not seen for well-child visits at this cadence, or at all. In the United States, public and private health insurance programs cover preventive well-child visits; however, families may struggle to attend appointments for other reasons (i.e., scheduling or transportation challenges, lack of awareness of the recommended visit schedule). Families of color, those with public health insurance or no insurance, and those living in rural locations are particularly likely to face barriers that make it difficult for them to access care.[2,3]

Costs of additional care can substantially affect the quality and timeliness of other needed healthcare for newborns and infants. Outside of well-child visits, the cost of healthcare can vary significantly depending on insurance coverage, the types of providers available, and needed care. This includes sick visits or follow-up for something potentially identified in a well-child visit with a specialist or the pediatrician. For many families, a lack of regular preventive care or availability of providers means that they must rely on the emergency department for minor health concerns.[4]

It is also recommended that infants have their first dental visit before they turn one year old.[5] One study found that as many as two-thirds of American families may not know of or follow through on this recommendation, in large part because they believe their baby's teeth are healthy. This data suggests a need for additional parent education around this topic.[6]

Just as it is important for parents to have personal healthcare providers they trust, it is equally important for parents to feel comfortable, heard, and respected in their relationships with their babies' healthcare providers. This is especially true for families of color, families with low socioeconomic resources, and other groups that have historically experienced challenges and barriers in the healthcare system. For families whose infants have complex medical needs continuous care with a trusted provider is also critical.[7]

Vaccinations

Leading health organizations have long advised that it is both safe and important for infants to be vaccinated against a range of serious and sometimes fatal diseases (i.e., polio, RSV, Hepatitis B, and more).[8] The vaccination schedule recommended by the American Academy of Pediatrics begins at birth and typically continues throughout future well-child visits.

Research has shown that parents learn about vaccinations from a variety of sources, such as their children's pediatrician, family and community members, the internet, and social media.[9] In recent years, there has been an uptick in parents delaying or refusing recommended vaccinations for their children.[10] Common reasons include religious beliefs, personal or philosophical beliefs, safety concerns, and a desire to obtain more information.[10,11] In one study, American parents who were hesitant about vaccinating their children reported that they began thinking about this topic before their children were born and that their beliefs had evolved over time. While parents in this study generally trusted their children's pediatricians, they did not believe they provided balanced information about the risks and benefits of vaccination.[12] These findings point to the importance of parents receiving accurate information and evidence-based guidance about infant vaccinations from healthcare, community, and social service providers who they trust.

Putting It Into Practice

- ***Provide anticipatory guidance about the importance of healthcare for newborns and infants.*** As a community or social service provider, you can help families to understand the importance of regular healthcare during the first year of life – including well-child visits and timely care when issues or illness arise. You can begin to discuss this topic before the baby is even born, link families to any needed healthcare resources (i.e., insurance coverage, local pediatricians), and help them to navigate complex healthcare systems.
- ***Talk with families about infant vaccinations and refer them to reputable sources of information on this topic.*** It is important that families have conversations with trusted partners about vaccination and access to reliable information about how vaccines work, the potential risks and benefits, and how they relate to a broader global public health strategy. Parents may mistakenly believe that they do not need to vaccinate their children because certain diseases (i.e., polio) are currently rare, not recognizing how growing rates of non-vaccination can actually increase the risk for their child and others.
- ***Monitor developmental milestones.*** Many community and social service providers engage in developmental monitoring and screenings of infants, including the use of validated screening instruments and tools. Developmental monitoring tracks development over time and helps to identify infants who may be experiencing developmental delays and in need of additional intervention.

- ***Ask how well-child visits are going, and support follow-up.*** You can check in regularly with families about scheduling well-child visits and follow-up to see how they went. You can listen when families have concerns about their child's health or their healthcare provider, working with them around communication and advocacy strategies so that their concerns are heard. With families' permission, you can also reach out to healthcare providers on their behalf to share screening results and professional observations.

Breastfeeding

Key Terms

Lactation: The bodily process of producing human milk.
Breastfeeding: The act of feeding a baby with human milk, either at the breast or with pumped milk.

Pooja's Story ♥

Pooja, a 22-year-old Indian-American woman, had given birth to a healthy baby boy two weeks ago. As a teenager, Pooja was molested by her uncle and turned to alcohol use as a coping mechanism. A few years later, she met her boyfriend and became pregnant. Upon seeing the positive test, she was determined to do everything she could to have a healthy pregnancy. With the support of her boyfriend and a counselor, she successfully abstained from alcohol for all nine months. During that time, she also learned about the benefits of breastfeeding, and decided that this was something she wanted to do.

Now, two weeks after giving birth, Pooja's son was a vigorous eater who seemed to want to breastfeed all the time, day and night. Whenever he latched, Pooja felt physically and emotionally overwhelmed, like she was having a panic attack. While she continued to avoid alcohol, she was beginning to have strong cravings for it again. She did not know what to do or where to turn for help. She did not have any female relatives close by, and she was the first of her friends to have a baby. Her counselor did not know much about breastfeeding, and her doctors only seemed to care that the baby was gaining weight. She wanted to continue breastfeeding, but was not sure if she could.

WHO and the American Academy of Pediatrics recommend that most babies should be exclusively breastfed for at least the first six months of life, and ideally up until 2 years of age.[13,14] Early and exclusive breastfeeding is associated with positive health outcomes – immediate and across the life course – for both parents and infants. Despite these health benefits, there are many disparities in breastfeeding initiation, length, and exclusivity across different groups in the United States. It is important for community and social service providers to understand some of the factors that may influence breastfeeding, and ways that they can support positive breastfeeding experiences for the families that they work with.

Importantly, the intention of the following discussion is to prepare community and social service providers to support families who are open to breastfeeding or interested in learning about it. There are many reasons why a parent may not breastfeed – from the parent or baby being physically unable to breastfeed, to logistical challenges (like having to go back to work or not having an adequate space to pump), to breastfeeding not being common in their family or culture, to simply not wanting to for personal or emotional reasons. Every parent's and family's choice should be respected, and no one should be pressured into breastfeeding if it is not right for them. In the end, "fed is best" – whether baby is fed at the breast, with pumped milk, or with formula.

Benefits

Decades of research has linked breastfeeding to positive health outcomes in both the short and long terms.[15] Notably, while these benefits are strongest when breastfeeding starts early in life and is exclusive (i.e., no supplementation with formula), even lower amounts of breastfeeding can have positive effects.[16] Researchers have found that when infants drink any amount of breastmilk for at least two months, their risk of SIDS is cut in half. Breastfeeding also strengthens infants' immune systems, making them less susceptible to ear, respiratory, and gastrointestinal infections.[15] In the longer term, research has also linked breastfeeding to better cognitive, language, and social-emotional skills, and lower rates of asthma, obesity, and diabetes.[16,17,18] Breastfeeding has also been linked to many short- and long-term maternal health benefits, and for the attachment relationship.[15,17,18]

Breastfeeding Disparities

Despite the many benefits of breastfeeding, there is evidence of significant disparities in breastfeeding during the first year of life.[19] In the United States, research has suggested that Black mothers face numerous barriers to breastfeeding, including lower knowledge or exposure to breastfeeding, limited social and healthcare support, financial costs related to pumping or obtaining lactation support, and challenges related to juggling breastfeeding and employment.[18,20,21,22] Breastfeeding disparities have also been found among Latina mothers depending on their level of acculturation. One study found that Spanish-speaking Latinas were more likely to breastfeed than predominately English-speaking Latinas, but that both groups were less likely to breastfeed than non-Latinas.[23] Breastfeeding rates have also found to be lower in neighborhoods that are more socioeconomically disadvantaged and that have fewer lactation resources, as well as among those who are younger or have less than a high school diploma.[15,24,25,26] These and other findings all point to the importance of tailoring interventions to families' unique social and cultural contexts.[27]

Across groups, cultural beliefs, knowledge about breastfeeding, and parental self-efficacy all influence families' decisions around breastfeeding.[28,29,30,31,32] Research has also demonstrated that stressors, trauma, and mental health can play a role in starting and continuing breastfeeding.[33] Women with histories of sexual abuse, intimate partner violence, and/or substance use disorders sometimes experience strong emotional and physical reactions while breastfeeding, which can result in discontinuation.[34,35] Other work has found that mothers who experienced at least one major stressor in the year before having a baby were less likely to start breastfeeding, and that those who did start were more likely to stop within four weeks. This was particularly true among mothers who had experienced emotional stressors or traumatic events.[36] Other findings have indicated that women who experienced depression before getting pregnant and/or during the postpartum period are less likely to breastfeed.[37,38]

Research has also demonstrated that social and economic stressors can result in early discontinuation of breastfeeding. One study of American mothers receiving public nutrition support found that food insecurity was a significant predictor of stopping breastfeeding.[39] Other groups that may be more likely to stop breastfeeding early include younger parents, those with lower levels of education, those who are single, those struggling with low milk supply, those with no prior breastfeeding experience, those who have to return to work within three months of giving birth, those with lower control over their jobs, and non-Hispanic Black parents.[40,41,42] On the other hand, higher levels of social support have been linked to longer durations of breastfeeding.[43]

Lactation Support and Other Interventions

Given the previously described benefits and disparities in breastfeeding, it is important for healthcare, community, and social service providers to be prepared to support families who want to breastfeed. It is also important that providers are mindful of any potential biases they may have around breastfeeding or formula feeding. Researchers have found that when providers are supportive toward breastfeeding, their clients are more likely to start breastfeeding and to have positive experiences. On the other hand, when providers are unsupportive or exhibit biased beliefs or behaviors around this topic, breastfeeding is less likely.[44,45]

There are numerous successful interventions to support breastfeeding and reduce disparities. During hospital deliveries, rooming in (when baby stays in the parent's room instead of a nursery), skin-to-skin contact, and early initiation of breastfeeding have all been found to promote higher rates of breastfeeding.[46,47,48,49] Education about breastfeeding and milk supply has also been found to be beneficial.[50] One study found that about 50% of American mothers supplement breast milk with formula because they believe that they are not making enough milk. While supplementation is sometimes appropriate, the team behind this study concluded that many parents would benefit from receiving education on infants' nutritional needs, how to identify true milk insufficiency, and how to obtain professional lactation support.[15] Support from a lactation professional can be helpful not only for addressing milk supply, but also for promoting breastfeeding parents' knowledge and confidence around other issues, such as breastfeeding and pumping techniques and schedules, latching issues, pain, breastfeeding an infant who is preterm or has health problems, and more.[51,52,53,54,55,56,57]

The knowledge and support of one's partner and/or support system can also have a large impact on breastfeeding outcomes. These individuals can support breastfeeding parents by physically helping the baby to latch, providing emotional support, and managing other household tasks – including care of other children – while the parent is breastfeeding. Studies have demonstrated that parents who have supportive partners are more likely to reach their breastfeeding goals, lifting up the importance of interventions and support professionals including partners in their conversations about breastfeeding.[58,59]

Breastfeeding expectations and experiences can also affect self-confidence and mental health during the postpartum period.[60] One study of predominately White women found that those whose breastfeeding experiences were going differently than they imagined when they were pregnant were more likely to report depression symptoms.[61] Therefore, lactation and social support are important not only for promoting breastfeeding, but for protecting the mental health and well-being of those who are breastfeeding.

Putting It Into Practice

- ***Explore feeding options.*** As noted earlier in this chapter, many community and social service providers begin working with families during pregnancy. This provides multiple opportunities to discuss options for feeding their baby and the benefits associated with breastfeeding. The safe, trusted relationship that families have with you may help them process complex feelings and reactions to different feeding options, as they know you will not judge them. Including partners in these conversations can also help families to reach their goals.
- ***Check in with the family soon after delivery.*** It can be helpful to make a plan with the family to check in soon after they arrive home with the infant. This can be beneficial for many reasons, including supporting the family around their feeding plan. For example, breastfeeding can often be very challenging, even if it seemed to be going smoothly while in the hospital or other birth setting. In addition to helping to ensure that the family receives help from a lactation support resource quickly, you can provide emotional support and reassurance during this stressful time.
- ***Help breastfeeding families to obtain necessary materials.*** As a community or social service provider, you can help ensure that those who are feeding their child breastmilk have access to needed materials, such as a breast pump. In the United States, most insurance providers cover breast pumps, but exact details vary and the logistics of obtaining a pump can be complicated. Manual breast pumps may also be available at the hospital, if families ask for one before they leave. You can also support families in accessing financial assistance for other needed materials (i.e., replacement pump parts, bottles).
- ***Ensure that breastfeeding parents know their rights.*** Encourage clients to inquire about their workplace policies around breastfeeding and pumping before they give birth to ensure that they know what their rights are and if there is anything they need to do in advance to ensure that supports are in place. Ensure that they are aware of breastfeeding protections in the workplace and support them in advocating for the fulfillment of these protections if they are not being honored. In the United States, the Fair Labor Standards Act that was passed in 2022 provides legal guidance for the rights of pumping parents, including adequate time and space to pump.
- ***Attend to the mental health of breastfeeding clients.*** As mentioned earlier, when breastfeeding experiences go differently than one imagined when pregnant, this can lead to symptoms of depression. As a community or social service provider, you should pay close attention to how your clients seem to be functioning and feeling, screen for depression and anxiety, and help them connect to mental health resources if needed. You will find suggestions throughout this book on strategies to employ when the availability of mental health services is limited in your community.

Community Baby Showers Δ

In Kansas, the Harvey County PAT Program and Chaparral Schools Unified School District (USD) 361 have partnered with the KIDS Network to host Community Baby Showers specifically for rural, low-resource areas, where access to prenatal and postpartum resources is often limited. These events provide an engaging environment for families, blending education with celebration to make learning accessible and enjoyable. Topics covered include the following.

- **Safe Sleep Practices**: Safe sleep guidance helps parents create a sleep environment that reduces the risk of SUID, emphasizing crib safety, sleep positioning, and more.
- **Tobacco Avoidance**: Expectant families learn about the risks of tobacco exposure during pregnancy and infancy, receiving encouragement and resources to quit smoking or minimize exposure.
- **Perinatal Mental Health**: These events highlight the importance of perinatal mental well-being, educating families on perinatal mood and anxiety disorders, and other mental health issues, while connecting them to community support.
- **Breastfeeding Education**: Families receive information on the benefits of breastfeeding and tips to overcome common challenges, equipping them with knowledge to make informed feeding choices.

To support the educational aspect, these events also include practical giveaways like safety-approved portable cribs, wearable blankets, car seats, diapers, humidifiers, air purifiers, and "goody bags" with baby care essentials. These items not only help alleviate the financial burden of new parenthood but also ensure that families have access to the tools they need for their babies' health and safety.

The atmosphere of these Community Baby Showers is vibrant and welcoming, with food, treats, and photo booth stations creating a festive and family-friendly environment. Personnel at the event guide families on how to access vital community resources, such as lactation support services and WIC, to ensure they know where to turn for ongoing help. The goal is to create a point of entry for maternal/child health services, energize families, boost their confidence, and foster a sense of readiness as they prepare to welcome a new baby. By providing practical tools and health education in a celebratory setting, these Safe Sleep Community Baby Showers empower families to care for their babies with confidence and lower the incidence of infant mortality.

For more information on these programs and their community baby showers, visit <www.cooper.usd373.org/services/parents-as-teachers> and <www.usd361.org>.

Brooke's Story With SJRC Texas PAT Δ

The SJRC Texas PAT program plays a critical role in supporting maternal and infant health by providing a network of specialized services that address the complex needs of families during the perinatal period – the time before and after a baby's birth.

This period is essential for both maternal and infant health, as it sets the stage for long-term well-being. Recognizing this, the SJRC Texas PAT program has implemented a series of focused initiatives and partnerships to address common issues that can impact maternal and infant morbidity and mortality.

Following are a few of the services offered by SJRC Texas PAT program.

1. **Mothers and Babies Certification for Parent Educators**: By training parent educators in the Mothers and Babies program, SJRC equips its staff to help parents manage stress and improve mental health during pregnancy and postpartum. This training is crucial because mental health challenges, including depression and anxiety, can affect both maternal and infant health outcomes.
2. **Safe Sleep Training Through Cribs for Kids**: With safe sleep training, SJRC aims to reduce risks associated with SIDS and other sleep-related deaths, which are significant contributors to infant mortality. This training ensures that parents receive guidance on creating safe sleeping environments for their babies, including recommendations on sleep position, crib setup, and room sharing.
3. **Breastfeeding Peer and Lactation Counseling**: SJRC's partnerships with breastfeeding peer counselors and certified lactation counselors provide essential support to new mothers, helping them establish and sustain breastfeeding behaviors. Breastfeeding has well-documented benefits for both mothers and infants, including lower risks of infections, chronic conditions, and improved maternal bonding, all of which positively affect maternal and infant morbidity and mortality rates.
4. **Access to Local Therapy Resources**: For families facing additional challenges, SJRC connects them with local therapy resources. This support can address mental health issues, developmental concerns, and stressors that may arise from economic or social circumstances, helping to reduce stress-related complications that affect maternal and infant health.
5. **Infant Massage Instruction**: Infant massage promotes bonding between parents and babies, and it can also improve an infant's emotional and physical health. This practice has been associated with benefits such as enhanced sleep, better digestion, and reduced stress responses in infants, all of which contribute to healthy development and well-being.

Through these services, the SJRC Texas PAT program aims to provide a comprehensive perinatal support system. This approach goes beyond immediate medical needs, addressing mental, emotional, and practical challenges that families face during this critical period. By proactively addressing factors that contribute to maternal and infant morbidity and mortality, SJRC offers families a foundation for healthier lives.

Notably, SJRC Texas has partnered with La Leche League to offer a "Breastfeeding and Pumping Support Group" through which new and expectant mothers gain access to breastfeeding advocacy, training, and emotional support. This support system has been transformative for families like Brooke's, a mother living in a rural Texas county with minimal local resources for breastfeeding support.

The support group connected Brooke with an International Board-Certified Lactation Consultant (IBCLC) who provided critical insight into her daughter Joanne's feeding issues. After discovering that a drop in Brooke's milk supply had caused Joanne to lose weight, the IBCLC offered guidance on increasing the milk supply. Within a week of implementing these strategies, Joanne's weight rebounded, putting her back on a healthy track. Additionally, Brooke accessed donor milk to support Joanne's nutritional needs and enrolled in an infant massage class, which further contributed to Joanne's health and well-being.

Reflecting on her experience, Brooke shared,

> Luckily, with some amazing women in my life who provide donor milk, we were able to get my daughter back to a healthy weight, and she is so much happier! I was able to breastfeed for 5½ months, and I am so grateful to my body for giving my baby what she needed for those five months."

Brooke's journey exemplifies the impact of community-based breastfeeding support, which can make a profound difference for families, especially those in underserved areas.

Through the dedicated efforts of the PAT program and the support of her community, Brooke and Joanne are thriving. Stories like theirs highlight the essential role that accessible breastfeeding support, education, and advocacy play in fostering healthy outcomes for mothers and babies.

For more information on the SJRC Texas PAT program and the perinatal services it provides, visit <www.sjrctexas.org>.

Your Role as a Community or Social Service Provider

Listening and Learning

The data and information in this chapter present a picture of both the importance of and challenges to consistent healthcare in the first year of life. Understanding the data, statistics, and stories specific to your community will help you to tailor your services to the issues, needs, and strengths of your local community and the families within it. Consider: what do you already know about the landscape of pediatric healthcare in your local community? (i.e., notable areas of strength, levels of cultural responsivity, presence of specialized care)? How can you learn more (i.e., researching information and local data, listening to personal stories of different kinds of families in your community)?

Advocating

As discussed earlier in this book, your role as a community or service provider operates on two levels: (a) your individual work with families; and (b) your work with systems, including local healthcare systems and providers. The information in this chapter pertains to both levels of work and also points to the need for broader advocacy for: (a) pediatric healthcare that truly partners with families; and (b) community and workplace environments that are supportive of breastfeeding. You can advocate within your organization – for example, by working to establish coordination agreements with clinics and providers that facilitate timely access to pediatric healthcare for families you work with; and for private, pleasant spaces for pumping and breastfeeding at your workplace. You can also advocate outside of your organization in the community at large by lifting up policies, programs, and initiatives that expand high-quality, culturally responsive pediatric healthcare services, as well as community environments and resources that support breastfeeding.

Take Time to Reflect

Reflecting on the practice implications throughout this chapter and your role as a community or social service provider, what is one area where you believe you are already doing an excellent job? What is one area where you could improve your professional practice or deepen your knowledge and understanding?

Take Action

Now that you have reflected on an area where you could improve your professional practice, create a SMART goal to make it happen. Remember, a SMART goal is described as follows.

- **S**pecific
- **M**easurable
- **A**chievable
- **R**elevant
- **T**ime-Bound

For example, imagine that you do not know much about lactation support services in your local area. A SMART goal might be:

> Many of my clients breastfeed and might benefit from lactation support (**Relevant**). Today (**Time-Bound**), I will set a timer for ten minutes and spend some conducting online searches for lactation consultants and support groups in my area. I hope to make a list of at least three resources I can share with my clients (**Specific, Achievable, Measurable**).

Key Takeaways From This Chapter

1. Regular healthcare and routine vaccinations are important to ensuring infants' healthy growth and development in the first year of life; however, many families face barriers and challenges in these domains.
2. Breastfeeding is associated with a range of benefits for infants' short- and long-term health, but breastfeeding rates are lower among some groups (i.e., Black families, those with lower socioeconomic resources, those struggling with depression) due to a variety of factors.

3. Lactation support and community-based interventions can play a significant role in supporting healthcare access, breastfeeding, and healthy outcomes for infants in the first year of life.

References

1. American Academy of Pediatrics (2023). *AAP schedule of well-child care visits.* www.healthychildren.org/English/family-life/health-management/Pages/Well-Child-Care-A-Check-Up-for-Success.aspx
2. Aloe, C. F., Hall, K. L., Pérez-Escamilla, R., Rosenthal, M. S., Fenick, A. M., & Sharifi, M. (2023). Multilevel factors associated with participation in group well-child care. *Academic Pediatrics, 23*(7), 1376–1384. https://doi.org/10.1016/j.acap.2023.03.004
3. Fuller, M. G., Lu, T., Gray, E. E., Jocson, M. A. L., Barger, M. K., Bennett, M., Lee, H. C., & Hintz, S. R. (2023). Rural residence and factors associated with attendance at the second high-risk infant follow-up clinic visit for very low birth weight infants in California. *American Journal of Perinatology, 40*(5), 546–556. https://doi.org/10.1055/s-0041-1729889
4. Jones, D. S., McNagny, S. E., Williams, M. V., Parker, R. M., Sawyer, M. F., & Rask, K. J. (1999). Lack of a regular source of care among children using a public hospital emergency department. *Pediatric Emergency Care, 15*(1), 13–16. https://doi.org/10.1097/00006565-199902000-00004
5. American Academy of Pediatric Dentistry (n.d.). *The importance of the age one dental visit.* www.aapd.org/globalassets/media/policy-center/year1visit.pdf
6. Yun, Q., Liu, M., Zhao, M., Yang, L., Miao, J., & Chang, C. (2022). The willingness to attend the first dental visit within 1 year of age: An analysis applying Andersen's behavioral model of health service utilization. *International Journal of Paediatric Dentistry, 32*(3), 324–333. https://doi.org/10.1111/ipd.12888
7. Kharrat, A., Moore, G. P., Beckett, S., Nicholls, S. G., Sampson, M., & Daboval, T. (2018). Antenatal consultations at extreme prematurity: A systematic review of parent communication needs. *The Journal of Pediatrics, 196*, 109–115. https://doi.org/10.1016/j.jpeds.2017.10.067
8. Centers for Disease Control and Prevention (2024). *About vaccines for your child.* www.cdc.gov/vaccines-children/about/index.html. Accessed December 2024.
9. Chung, Y., Schamel, J., Fisher, A., & Frew, P. M. (2017). Influences on immunization decision-making among US parents of young children. *Maternal and Child Health Journal, 21*(12), 2178–2187. https://doi.org/10.1007/s10995-017-2336-6
10. Novilla, M. L. B., Goates, M. C., Redelfs, A. H., Quenzer, M., Novilla, L. K. B., Leffler, T., Holt, C. A., Doria, R. B., Dang, M. T., Hewitt, M., Lind, E., Prickett, E., & Aldridge, K. (2023). Why parents say no to having their children vaccinated against measles: A systematic review of the social determinants of parental perceptions on MMR vaccine hesitancy. *Vaccines, 11*(5), 926. https://doi.org/10.3390/vaccines11050926
11. McKee, C., & Bohannon, K. (2016). Exploring the reasons behind parental refusal of vaccines. *The Journal of Pediatric Pharmacology and Therapeutics, 21*(2), 104–109. https://doi.org/10.5863/1551-6776-21.2.104
12. Glanz, J. M., Wagner, N. M., Narwaney, K. J., Shoup, J. A., McClure, D. L., McCormick, E. V., & Daley, M. F. (2013). A mixed methods study of parental vaccine decision making and parent-provider trust. *Academic Pediatrics, 13*(5), 481–488. https://doi.org/10.1016/j.acap.2013.05.030
13. World Health Organization (n.d.). *Breastfeeding.* www.who.int/health-topics/breastfeeding#tab=tab_1
14. Centers for Disease Control and Prevention (2024). *Breastfeeding: Recommendations and benefits.* www.cdc.gov/nutrition/infantandtoddlernutrition/breastfeeding/recommendations-benefits.html
15. Lessen, R., & Kavanagh, K. (2015). Position of the Academy of Nutrition and Dietetics: Promoting and supporting breastfeeding. *Journal of the Academy of Nutrition and Dietetics, 115*(3), 444–449. https://doi.org/10.1016/j.jand.2014.12.014

16. Khan, J., Vesel, L., Bahl, R., & Martines, J. C. (2015). Timing of breastfeeding initiation and exclusivity of breastfeeding during the first month of life: Effects on neonatal mortality and morbidity – a systematic review and meta-analysis. *Maternal and Child Health Journal*, *19*(3), 468–479. https://doi.org/10.1007/s10995-014-1526-8
17. Krol, K. M., & Grossmann, T. (2018). Psychological effects of breastfeeding on children and mothers. *Bundesgesundheitsblatt-Gesundheitsforschung-Gesundheitsschutz*, *61*(8), 977–985. https://doi.org/10.1007/s00103-018-2769-0
18. Beauregard, J. L., Hamner, H. C., Chen, J., Avila-Rodriguez, W., Elam-Evans, L. D., & Perrine, C. G. (2019). Racial disparities in breastfeeding initiation and duration among US infants born in 2015. *Morbidity and Mortality Weekly Report*, *68*(34), 745. https://doi.org/10.15585/mmwr.mm6834a3 10.15585/mmwr.mm6834a3. Accessed December 2024.
19. Chung, E. K., Painter, I., Sitcov, K., & Souter, V. D. (2022). Exclusive breastfeeding in the Northwest: Disparities related to race/ethnicity and substance use. *Academic Pediatrics*, *22*(6), 918–926. https://doi.org/10.1016/j.acap.2021.09.016
20. Hinson, T. D., Skinner, A. C., & Spatz, D. L. (2021). Subject matter experts identify health equity concerns in breastfeeding for African American women. *The Journal of Perinatal & Neonatal Nursing*, *35*(2), 160–168. https://doi.org/10.1097/JPN.0000000000000486
21. Scott, A., & Kirkland, T. (2023). Rethinking breastfeeding management: A patient-centered approach based on new guidelines. *The Nurse Practitioner*, *48*(3), 11–19. https://doi.org/10.1097/01.NPR.0000000000000012
22. Sartor, L., Pyram-Vincent, C., Lin, H. M., Ouyang, Y., Wax, D. B., & Beilin, Y. (2024). Race and intention to breastfeed are the strongest predictors of exclusive breastfeeding: A retrospective study. *Journal of Racial and Ethnic Health Disparities*, *11*(6), 3704–3713. https://doi.org/10.1007/s40615-023-01819-8
23. Sebastian, R. A., Coronado, E., Otero, M. D., McKinney, C. R., & Ramos, M. M. (2019). Associations between maternity care practices and 2-month breastfeeding duration vary by race, ethnicity, and acculturation. *Maternal and Child Health Journal*, *23*(6), 858–867. https://doi.org/10.1007/s10995-018-02711-2
24. Butler, M. S., Smart, B. P., Watson, E. J., Narla, S. S., & Keenan-Devlin, L. (2023). U.S. breastfeeding outcomes at the intersection: Differences in duration among racial and ethnic groups with varying educational attainment in a nationally representative sample. *Journal of Human Lactation*, *39*(4), 722–732. https://doi.org/10.1177/08903344231186786
25. Kopp, S. J., Kelly, E. A., & DeFranco, E. A. (2023). Influence of social determinants of health on breastfeeding intent in the United States. *Birth*, *50*(4), 858–867. https://doi.org/10.1111/birt.12740
26. Yourkavitch, J., Kane, J. B., & Miles, G. (2018). Neighborhood disadvantage and neighborhood affluence: Associations with breastfeeding practices in urban areas. *Maternal and Child Health Journal*, *22*(4), 546–555. https://doi.org/10.1007/s10995-017-2423-8
27. Stevens-Watkins, D., Hargons, C. N., Dogan, J., Malone, N., Jester, J. K., Thorpe, S., & Linares, A. M. (2022). Social health care determinants of breastfeeding Black women: A multigenerational study. *Breastfeeding Medicine*, *17*(8), 666–672. https://doi.org/10.1089/bfm.2021.0258
28. Quintero, S. M., Strassle, P. D., Londoño Tobón, A., Ponce, S., Alhomsi, A., Maldonado, A. I., Ko, J. S., Wilkerson, M. J., & Nápoles, A. M. (2023). Race/ethnicity-specific associations between breastfeeding information source and breastfeeding rates among U.S. women. *BMC Public Health*, *23*(1), 520. https://doi.org/10.1186/s12889-023-15447-8
29. Zhang, Q., Lamichhane, R., Wouk, K., Guthrie, J., & Li, K. (2021). Prenatal perception of breastfeeding recommendations predicts early breastfeeding outcomes of participants in the Special Supplemental Nutrition Program for Women, Infants, and Children (WIC). *The American Journal of Clinical Nutrition*, *114*(6), 1949–1959. https://doi.org/10.1093/ajcn/nqab268
30. Korth, C. X., Keim, S. A., Crerand, C. E., & Jackson, J. L. (2022). New mothers' perceptions of pressure to breastfeed. *MCN. The American Journal of Maternal Child Nursing*, *47*(3), 160–167. https://doi.org/10.1097/NMC.0000000000000814
31. Alghamdi, S., Horodynski, M., & Stommel, M. (2017). Racial and ethnic differences in breastfeeding, maternal knowledge, and self-efficacy among low-income mothers. *Applied Nursing Research*, *37*, 24–27. https://doi.org/10.1016/j.apnr.2017.07.009

32. Rosenthal, A., Oliveira, S. B., Madubuko, U., Tanuos, H., Schwab, J., & Monteiro, I. M. (2019). Effects of immigration on infant feeding practices in an inner city, low socioeconomic community. *Journal of the National Medical Association*, *111*(2), 153–157. https://doi.org/10.1016/j.jnma.2018.07.006
33. Dugat, V. M., Chertok, I. R. A., & Haile, Z. T. (2019). Association between stressful life events and exclusive breastfeeding among mothers in the United States. *Breastfeeding Medicine*, *14*(7), 475–481. https://doi.org/10.1089/bfm.2019.0058
34. Jansson, L. M., Velez, M. L., & Butz, A. M. (2017). The effect of sexual abuse and prenatal substance use on successful breastfeeding. *Journal of Obstetric, Gynecologic & Neonatal Nursing*, *46*(3), 480–484. https://doi.org/10.1016/j.jogn.2017.02.002
35. Ribeiro, M. R. C., Batista, R. F. L., Schraiber, L. B., Pinheiro, F. S., Santos, A. M. D., Simões, V. M. F., Confortin, S. C., Aristizabal, L. Y. G., Yokokura, A. V. C. P., & Silva, A. A. M. D. (2021). Recurrent violence, violence with complications, and intimate partner violence against pregnant women and breastfeeding duration. *Journal of Women's Health (2002)*, *30*(7), 979–989. https://doi.org/10.1089/jwh.2020.8378
36. Kitsantas, P., Gaffney, K. F., Nirmalraj, L., & Sari, M. (2019). The influence of maternal life stressors on breastfeeding outcomes: A US population-based study. *The Journal of Maternal-Fetal & Neonatal Medicine*, *32*(11), 1869–1873. https://doi.org/10.1080/14767058.2017.1421929
37. Wallenborn, J. T., Joseph, A. C., Graves, W. C., & Masho, S. W. (2018). Prepregnancy depression and breastfeeding duration: A look at maternal age. *Journal of Pregnancy*, *2018*. https://doi.org/10.1155/2018/4825727
38. Wouk, K., Stuebe, A. M., & Meltzer-Brody, S. (2017). Postpartum mental health and breastfeeding practices: An analysis using the 2010–2011 Pregnancy Risk Assessment Monitoring System. *Maternal and Child Health Journal*, *21*(3), 636–647. https://doi.org/10.1007/s10995-016-2150-6
39. Gallo, S., Kogan, K., & Kitsantas, P. (2019). Racial and ethnic differences in reasons for breastfeeding cessation among women participating in the Special Supplemental Nutrition Program for Women, Infants, and Children. *Journal of Midwifery & Women's Health*, *64*(6), 725–733. https://doi.org/10.1111/jmwh.13031
40. Rozga, M. R., Kerver, J. M., & Olson, B. H. (2015). Self-reported reasons for breastfeeding cessation among low-income women enrolled in a peer counseling breastfeeding support program. *Journal of Human Lactation*, *31*(1), 129–137. https://doi.org/10.1177/0890334414548070
41. Hamner, H. C., Chiang, K. V., & Li, R. (2021). Returning to work and breastfeeding duration at 12 months, WIC infant and toddler feeding practices study-2. *Breastfeeding Medicine*, *16*(12), 956–964. https://doi.org/10.1089/bfm.2021.0081
42. Whitley, M. D., Ro, A., & Choi, B. (2022). Low job control and racial disparities in breastfeeding. *Journal of Occupational and Environmental Medicine*, *64*(8), e482–e491. https://doi.org/10.1097/JOM.0000000000002591
43. Lyons, G. C., Kay, M. C., Duke, N. N., Bian, A., Schildcrout, J. S., Perrin, E. M., Rothman, R. L., Yin, H. S., Sanders, L. M., Flower, K. B., Delamater, A. M., & Heerman, W. J. (2023). Social support and breastfeeding outcomes among a racially and ethnically diverse population. *American Journal of Preventive Medicine*, *64*(3), 352–360. https://doi.org/10.1016/j.amepre.2022.10.002
44. Berwick, M., & Louis-Jacques, A. F. (2023). Prenatal counseling and preparation for breastfeeding. *Obstetrics and Gynecology Clinics of North America*, *50*(3), 549–565. https://doi.org/10.1016/j.ogc.2023.03.007
45. Kendall-Tackett, K., & Moberg, K. U. (2018). Is it really mothers' choice? Systemic and provider barriers to breastfeeding. *Clinical Lactation*, *9*(4), 193–199. https://doi.org/10.1891/2158-0782.9.4.193
46. Augustyn, M., Haskins, D., Gross, S., Resnik, A. K., Ducharme-Smith, K., Orta-Aleman, D., Silbert-Flagg, J., Rosenblum, N., & Caulfield, L. E. (2023). Maternity care experiences and breastfeeding at discharge among Maryland WIC participants: A qualitative analysis. *Birth*, *50*(4), 1009–1017. https://doi.org/10.1111/birt.12758
47. Tully, K. P., Smith, J. L., Pearsall, M. S., Sullivan, C., Seashore, C., & Stuebe, A. M. (2022). Postnatal unit experiences associated with exclusive breastfeeding during the inpatient stay: A cross-sectional online survey. *Journal of Human Lactation*, *38*(2), 287–297. https://doi.org/10.1177/08903344211057876

48. Hemingway, S., Forson-Dare, Z., Ebeling, M., & Taylor, S. N. (2021). Racial disparities in sustaining breastfeeding in a baby-friendly designated southeastern United States hospital: An opportunity to investigate systemic racism. *Breastfeeding Medicine*, *16*(2), 150–155. https://doi.org/10.1089/bfm.2020.0306
49. Merewood, A., Bugg, K., Burnham, L., Krane, K., Nickel, N., Broom, S., Edwards, R., & Feldman-Winter, L. (2019). Addressing racial inequities in breastfeeding in the southern United States. *Pediatrics*, *143*(2). https://doi.org/10.1542/peds.2018-1897
50. Yesil, Y., Ekşioğlu, A., & Turfan, E. C. (2022). The effect of hospital-based breastfeeding group education given early perinatal period on breastfeeding self-efficacy and breastfeeding status. *Journal of Neonatal Nursing*, *29*(1), 81–90. https://doi.org/10.1016/j.jnn.2022.02.013
51. Schafer, E. J., Campo, S., Colaizy, T. T., Mulder, P. J., Breheny, P., & Ashida, S. (2017). First-time mothers' breast-feeding maintenance: Role of experiences and changes in maternal perceptions. *Public Health Nutrition*, *20*(17), 3099–3108. https://doi.org/10.1017/S136898001700221X
52. Bennett, C. F., Galloway, C., & Grassley, J. S. (2018). Education for WIC peer counselors about breastfeeding the late preterm infant. *Journal of Nutrition Education and Behavior*, *50*(2), 198–202. https://doi.org/10.1016/j.jneb.2017.05.364
53. Keenan-Devlin, L. S., Awosemusi, Y. F., Grobman, W., Simhan, H., Adam, E., Culhane, J., Miller, G., & Borders, A. E. (2019). Early term delivery and breastfeeding outcomes. *Maternal and Child Health Journal*, *23*(10), 1339–1347. https://doi.org/10.1007/s10995-019-02787-4
54. Omidi, A., Rahmani, S., Amini, R., & Karami, M. (2022). The effect of a planned lactation education program on the mother's breastfeeding practice and weight gain in low birth weight infants: A randomized clinical trial study. *BMC Pregnancy and Childbirth*, *22*(1), 482. https://doi.org/10.1186/s12884-022-04810-z
55. Furman, L., Feinstein, J., & Delozier, S. (2023). Understanding breastfeeding barriers at an urban pediatric practice. *Journal of Racial and Ethnic Health Disparities*, *10*(2), 581–592. https://doi.org/10.1007/s40615-022-01248-z
56. Louis-Jacques, A. F., Deubel, T. F., Vereen, S., Hernandez, I., Taylor, M., Miller, E. M., & Wilson, R. (2022). Doula perspectives on lactation education and breastfeeding support for diverse, low-income women: A field report. *Ecology of Food and Nutrition*, *61*(5), 638–648. https://doi.org/10.1080/03670244.2022.2116434
57. Keim, S. A., Jackson, J. L., Litteral, J. L., Schofield, K. A., & Crerand, C. E. (2021). Perceptions about lactation consultant support, breastfeeding experiences and postpartum psychosocial outcomes. *Maternal and Child Health Journal*, *25*(3), 497–506. https://doi.org/10.1007/s10995-020-03056-5
58. Ogbo, F. A., Akombi, B. J., Ahmed, K. Y., Rwabilimbo, A. G., Ogbo, A. O., Uwaibi, N. E., Ezeh, O. K., Agho, K. E., & On Behalf of the Global Maternal and Child Health Research Collaboration GloMACH (2020). Breastfeeding in the community-how can partners/fathers help? A systematic review. *International Journal of Environmental Research and Public Health*, *17*(2), 413. https://doi.org/10.3390/ijerph17020413
59. Gebremariam, K. T., Wynter, K., Zheng, M., Rawstorn, J. C., Denney-Wilson, E., & Laws, R. (2024). Breastfeeding – a survey of fathers' support needs and preferred sources of information. *International Breastfeeding Journal*, *19*(1), 50. https://doi.org/10.1186/s13006-024-00654-9
60. Elder, M., Murphy, L., Notestine, S., & Weber, A. (2022). Realigning expectations with reality: A case study on maternal mental health during a difficult breastfeeding journey. *Journal of Human Lactation*, *38*(1), 190–196. https://doi.org/10.1177/08903344211031142
61. Gregory, E. F., Butz, A. M., Ghazarian, S. R., Gross, S. M., & Johnson, S. B. (2015). Are unmet breastfeeding expectations associated with maternal depressive symptoms? *Academic Pediatrics*, *15*(3), 319–325. https://doi.org/10.1016/j.acap.2014.12.003

9 Supporting Healthy Lifestyles and Relationships

Self-Care Moment

A well-rounded diet is important fuel for the work that we do (and for reading long book chapters). Take a moment to check in with your body. Are you hungry? Are you craving anything? If so, what type of snack or meal would feel good and energizing to your body right now?

During pregnancy, one's health and lifestyle (i.e., around nutrition, sleep, exercise, and more) can directly affect the well-being of their baby, but living a healthy lifestyle can be challenging for any busy parent – particularly those from groups that experience challenges or barriers related to SDOH (i.e., access to affordable and nutritious food, eligibility for parental leave, exposure to stress or violence, exposure to pollution;).

Community and social service providers can make a difference by helping families explore aspects of a healthy lifestyle, navigate challenges and barriers, and set achievable goals. To this end, this chapter focuses on healthy lifestyle and relationship considerations during pregnancy and the postpartum period, including discussion of research on this topic, practice implications for your work, and reflections on your role as a community or social service provider. You will also hear the stories of Gianna and Abidemi, two pregnant women with very different struggles related to nutrition and weight gain during pregnancy; PAT's Healthy Eating and Active Living Taught in the Home (HEALTH) initiative; and Elena, a pregnant mother experiencing intimate partner violence.

Key Terms

Gestational weight gain: The amount of weight someone gains over the course of the pregnancy. The recommended amount of weight to gain during pregnancy depends on several factors, such as one's pre-pregnancy weight, health conditions, whether they are carrying multiples, and more.

Body mass index (BMI): Body mass index is a commonly used measurement of the ratio of a person's height to weight, intended to serve as an estimate of relative

DOI: 10.4324/9781003476474-9

body fat. In recent years, many medical experts have called BMI into question. For example, according to a policy from the American Medical Association (AMA)[1]:

> Due to significant limitations associated with the widespread use of BMI in clinical settings, the AMA suggests that it be used in conjunction with other valid measures of risk such as, but not limited to, measurements of visceral fat, body adiposity index, body composition, relative fat mass, waist circumference and genetic/metabolic factors . . . . The AMA also recognizes that relative body shape and composition differences across race/ethnic groups, sexes, genders, and age-span is essential to consider.

U.S. Institute of Medicine (IOM) recommendations: IOM recommendations are the guidelines provided by the U.S. Institute of Medicine (IOM). The recommendations provide defined clinical practice guidelines intended to optimize patient care and health outcomes.

Gestational diabetes: Gestational diabetes is a form of diabetes that occurs and is diagnosed during pregnancy (gestation). Like other types of diabetes, it affects how the body processes insulin. Gestational diabetes causes high blood sugar that can affect both maternal and infant health. It typically resolves after childbirth.

Folic Acid: Folic acid is a B vitamin that helps the body make healthy new cells. Everyone needs folic acid, but it is especially important for those who may get pregnant and who are pregnant. Getting enough folic acid before and during pregnancy can help to prevent birth defects of the brain and/or spine.

The "40-day rule," also known as postpartum confinement: A traditional practice in many cultures that calls for a 40-day period of physical rest to allow the postpartum individual to heal, bond with their baby, and relax.

Maternity leave or parental leave: A period of time during which parents are entitled to take off work to care for a newborn or adopted child without risk of losing their jobs. Policies vary widely across countries, regions, and companies regarding who is entitled to take parental leave and for how long.

Intimate partner violence (IPV): A pattern of physical and/or coercive behavior by someone who is, was, or wants to be in an intimate or dating relationship with someone. Examples include, but are not limited to, physical violence, emotional abuse, sexual assault, intimidation, and reproductive pressure.

Reproductive coercion: Coercive behavior in which one partner pressures, manipulates, tricks, interferes with, or threatens another into certain reproductive behavior (i.e., taking or not taking birth control, becoming pregnant, terminating a pregnancy).

Research Summary

Nutrition, Weight Management, Exercise, and Sleep

There are many personal, cultural, social, and other factors that influence eating habits, physical activity, and sleep patterns – before, during, and after pregnancy. For example, one study of pregnant and postpartum women found six key factors that support healthy lifestyles during pregnancy: (a) motivation to have a health pregnancy and baby and a quick postpartum recovery; (b) pre-pregnancy knowledge and experiences about what to expect during pregnancy and the postpartum period; (c) a desire to prioritize wellness during pregnancy and the postpartum period; (d) social support; (e) accountability; and (f) using technology to reinforce positive lifestyle changes.[2] Notably, each of these six factors are ones in which community and social service providers can make a difference – by providing education, helping clients to set goals, and providing referrals to other providers or resources that can help.

This subsection describes issues related to weight management, nutrition, exercise, and sleep that are important for community and social service providers to know about. Before diving in, it is important to acknowledge that these topics can be sensitive (i.e., focusing on weight gain/loss can be triggering for people with histories of disordered eating). While these topics should not be avoided, they should always be discussed respectfully and with sensitivity to personal and cultural factors.

Gianna's Story ♥

Gianna, a 25-year-old Italian American woman, was thrilled to be pregnant with her first baby, but nervous about the changes that would happen to her body. Gianna had struggled with her weight for most of her life and had tried many extreme diets over the years. Now that she was pregnant, her mother and grandmother were constantly bringing heaping trays of pasta and dessert to her house and serving her extra portions during meals. "You're eating for two! You don't want the baby to be too skinny!" they would say. Gianna knew they were well-intentioned, but the pressure and attention on her body made her feel uncomfortable.

Later, she went to a check-up at her midwife's office, and they asked her to step on the scale. Gianna had not weighed herself in several years because she knew that she would get stuck on the number, instead of focusing on her overall health and how her body felt. But before she could say anything, the nurse loudly announced her weight. Even though the nurse said she was right on track, it was still the heaviest she had been in a long time. She felt defeated and like she might cry.

Abidemi's Story ♥

Abidemi, a 35-year-old African woman living in an East Coast city, and her husband had two young sons when they learned they were expecting twins. The family lived in a one-bedroom apartment and was on the waitlist for a two-bedroom. Abidemi had recently been laid off from her job as a cashier, and her husband worked long hours as a janitor. They were doing their best to make ends meet despite a very tight budget. Groceries, in particular, were a hardship given rising costs and limited access to fresh produce in their neighborhood. Many days, Abidemi and her husband gave their sons the meat and produce they had on hand and ate smaller meals themselves. As Abidemi's pregnancy continued, she often felt tired and a bit lightheaded. At her second-trimester check-up, her doctor said that she was not gaining enough weight and that her iron levels were low.

Pre-Pregnancy Weight Management

Pre-pregnancy weight is a factor that can play a significant role in pregnancy outcomes.[3] It can influence pre-existing health conditions that may affect pregnancy and can also influence health outcomes after birth. Ideally, pre-pregnancy weight falls within the typical range for someone's height, however, this is not always the case. Weight management guidelines during pregnancy will vary depending on any specific concerns about pre-pregnancy weight. Notably, being either significantly under or over recommended weight ranges for one's height can pose health risks during pregnancy.[4]

Obesity prior to pregnancy is a significant risk factor for health problems/complications, and even death during pregnancy, childbirth, and the postpartum period. It is also closely related to SDOH (i.e., access to affordable, nutritious food; the local physical environment; exposure to stress; education). Research in the United States supports this connection, finding that Black and Latinx people, particularly those living in lower resource areas, are at increased risk for being overweight or obese.[5] The link between high pre-pregnancy BMI and increased risk of infant death held true even when those individuals kept their pregnancy weight gain within recommended ranges. In another study, researchers found a link between pre-pregnancy obesity and increased risk of stillbirth, which they said was likely due to a number of factors, such as abnormal placenta functioning, the presence of medical conditions such as diabetes, and hormonal, metabolic, and inflammatory imbalances related to obesity.[6] These findings point to the importance of preconception healthcare and supporting weight management before pregnancy whenever possible.

Gestational Weight Gain and Postpartum Weight Management

Gestational weight gain is a normal and important part of pregnancy. This weight gain reflects not only the size of the developing baby, but growth of the breasts and uterus, the development of the placenta and amniotic fluid, increased blood and fluid in the body, and increased fat stores.[7]

Research has found that many people do not have accurate knowledge of recommended weight gain during pregnancy.[8] Contrary to popular belief, recommended weight gain during pregnancy is not the same for everyone. Rather, it depends on several factors, such as pre-pregnancy BMI (despite the challenges of this measurement, as previously described) and whether someone is carrying multiples. The American College of Obstetricians and Gynecologists' recommendations for gestational weight gain are as follow.[9]

- "Underweight" pre-pregnancy BMI: Gain 28–40 pounds;
- "Normal" pre-pregnancy BMI: Gain 25–35 pounds, or 37–54 pounds if having twins;
- "Overweight" pre-pregnancy BMI: Gain 15–25 pounds, or 31–50 pounds if having twins; and
- "Obese" pre-pregnancy BMI: Gain 11–20 pounds, or 25–42 pounds if having twins.

While gaining adequate weight during pregnancy is important, there can be negative effects from gaining too much weight. Those whose gestational weight gain is above the recommended ranges are at increased risk for numerous health problems/complications, such as hypertension, gestational diabetes, breastfeeding complications, and postpartum weight retention and obesity.[10] Research has also documented a strong association between higher gestational weight gain and increased risk of complications during childbirth, including preterm delivery and C-section, as well as increased risk of stillbirth among those who are obese.[11] Meanwhile, gaining too little weight during pregnancy can also be problematic. Those who do not gain enough weight during pregnancy are at increased risk for preterm delivery, having babies who are low birthweight, and stillbirth.[11,12]

Overall, there are many social, cultural, and contextual factors that can influence weight gain during pregnancy – such as negative emotions, body image, discomfort, low energy, motivation, social support, and experiences of discrimination.[13,14] Several pre-pregnancy factors are also important – for example, pre-pregnancy weight, education and health literacy, medical conditions, mental health conditions, and history of disordered eating.[15,16] Notably, many of these factors are related to SDOH.

Weight management is also an important health topic during the postpartum period. Despite societal pressures to "bounce back" quickly after giving birth, it is important to recognize that postpartum healing takes many months, and that a variety of factors can affect that timeline (i.e., health problems/complications, breastfeeding). In the "fourth trimester," it is typically recommended to focus on good nutrition, rest, and light to moderate physical activity (rather than the numbers on the scale). However, over time, working toward an appropriate weight for one's body is important for reducing the risk of long-term health issues such as diabetes, heart disease, cancer, and future pregnancy complications.[17,18]

Nutrition and Exercise Before, During, and After Pregnancy

A balanced diet before, during, and after pregnancy is important for both maternal and infant health. This includes consuming a variety of nutritious foods (i.e., protein, fruits, vegetables, whole grains), which can look somewhat different across cultures. It also includes consuming an adequate (but not excessive) amount of calories. Contrary to the common belief that it is necessary to "eat for two," the American College of Obstetricians and Gynecologists advises that those who are pregnant with one baby only need an extra 340 calories per day starting in their second trimester, and slightly more than that in the third trimester.[19]

A variety of personal, cultural, and social factors affect nutrition and eating habits before, during, and after pregnancy.[20] For example, one study identified ten factors that influenced prenatal fruit and vegetable intake, including: (a) social support; (b) family structure; (c) access to fruits and vegetables; (d) food preferences; (e) knowledge about fruits and vegetables; (f) expectations about the health benefits of eating fruits and vegetables; (g) self-efficacy; (h) intentions; (i) action plans and coping strategies related to fruit and vegetable intake; and (j) maternal health. Social support from family/friends emerged as a primary factor driving fruit and vegetable consumption during pregnancy.[21]

Another study of primarily lower-income pregnant women with diabetes found that many participants did not feel confident or empowered in their ability to make changes to their diets. Specific barriers to good nutrition that were identified included: (a) feeling overwhelmed; (b) understanding and decoding nutrition labels; (c) managing nutrition choices in the context of food insecurity; (d) experiencing lack of control and motivation; (e) balancing dietary recommendations with preferences and cultural food norms; (f) maintaining a healthy eating schedule; and (g) integrating nutrition needs into family and social life. The authors of the study stressed the importance of culturally informed and practical nutrition supports that address the needs and constraints of those living in under-resourced communities.[22]

Exercise is another essential element of a healthy lifestyle and is generally considered safe during and after pregnancy with clearance from a healthcare provider.[23] Studies of those who exercised during pregnancy have shown outcomes such as lower rates of gestational hypertension and diabetes, shorter labors, lower rates of C-section, and shorter postpartum recovery times.[24,25,26,27,28] Physical activity also can be an essential factor in the prevention of depressive disorders in the postpartum period.[29,30,31,32] Despite these benefits, many individuals experience decreased motivation to exercise during pregnancy as their bodies and energy levels change.[33,34] Starting in the first weeks of pregnancy, many individuals also decrease how long, how often, and how intensely they exercise.[33] These findings point to the importance of reminding pregnant clients about the benefits of exercise and supporting their motivation and goal-setting in this area.[35]

Take Time to Reflect

From your perspective, what are some of the greatest challenges that your pregnant and postpartum clients face around nutrition and exercise? What are the greatest opportunities or motivators?

Supportive Interventions Around Nutrition, Exercise, and Weight Management During Pregnancy

Healthcare providers and clients alike often find it difficult or uncomfortable to talk about issues related to weight and nutrition – feelings which can be related to personal or cultural beliefs and experiences.[36,37] To this end, many people receive limited or inaccurate advice from both healthcare providers and family members about nutrition, weight gain, and maintaining a healthy lifestyle during pregnancy – despite the fact that they need and want information on these topics.[38,39,40,41,42,43,44] This is concerning, given that research has shown that when people receive accurate information and guidance, they are more likely to have healthy outcomes.[42]

Knowledgeable community and social service providers can play valuable roles in educating and supporting good nutrition, weight management, and exercise during pregnancy, and incorporating peer support has also been found to be helpful.[38,45] Such supports can be especially impactful for overweight or obese individuals who are thinking about getting pregnant, for those who were overweight or obese before pregnancy, for those who have previously had C-sections, and those experiencing postpartum depression, among others.[46,47] Notably, one study of individuals who were obese before pregnancy found that lack of nutritional knowledge was not the most significant factor that predicted eating habits and weight gain during pregnancy. Rather, food cravings, fatigue, nearby food options, feelings of self-efficacy, and lack of emotional and informational support were the biggest factors.[48] These findings underscore the importance of not only informational resources, but emotional support for those who are struggling around these issues during pregnancy.

Putting It Into Practice

- ***Recognize the complexities of weight management.*** Your relationship with and understanding of each family positions you to recognize and empathize with the specific complexities and barriers that can make healthy nutrition and exercise more challenging. This recognition and empathy can help decrease the resistance many people feel when talking about issues related to health and weight, opening space to identify small, achievable health-related goals. Further, you may be able to help your client explore how their health goals intersect with broader aspects of their parenting and/or life goals.

- ***Facilitate connections to nutrition resources.*** As a community or social service provider, you may also be able to facilitate connections to resources that can help your pregnant clients to reach their goals, including but not limited to income support and grocery assistance. Nutrition counseling and education may be particularly beneficial for individuals who have chronic and/or complex struggles with weight and body image. In the United States, families may be unaware that many private insurance providers cover nutrition counseling and education, as does Medicaid in several states.
- ***Incorporate nutrition-focused curricula or interventions.*** With additional training and resources, community and social service providers can embed nutritional curricula and/or interventions into their work with pregnant families. It is important that the selected curricula or interventions align with the values and overall mission of your work and fit with each family's individual context.

PAT's Healthy Eating and Active Living Taught in the Home (HEALTH) Initiative Δ

PAT has established a collaborative partnership with Washington University in St. Louis, Missouri to integrate a focus on healthy eating and active living into its home visiting model. This initiative, known as HEALTH, targets the prevention of diabetes and obesity, particularly in at-risk populations. Key contributors to this partnership include Dr. Debra Haire-Joshu, Dr. Rachel Tabak, and Cindy Schwarz, all of whom bring extensive experience in public health, behavioral science, nutrition and dietetics, and implementation science.

Through the 30-plus–year partnership, different iterations of health interventions have been tested within PAT across the United States. By incorporating HEALTH into PAT, home visitors are equipped to share culturally relevant, evidence-based strategies for nutritious eating and active living with families in a practical, supportive manner. This initiative is particularly aimed at pregnant women and young children, helping establish healthy habits early to reduce the risk of chronic conditions later in life.

Findings from these studies indicated positive outcomes for mothers and families in the PAT HEALTH program, including the following.

- Improved dietary intake, knowledge, and parental modeling.[49]
- Improved fruit and vegetable consumption and parents' improve food preparation skills.[49]
- Less weight gained weekly and total during gestation and through 12 months postpartum.[50,51]

- Reduced intake of soda and other sugar-sweetened beverages.[52]
- Increased physical activity.[52]
- Achievement of weight loss and reduced weight circumference.[52]

The health of mothers in the studies were improved, which can reduce their risk of preventable complications and death in the prenatal and postpartum space and promote long-lasting effects on maternal and family health. To date, the program has worked with 150 affiliates across the United States, involving over 3,000 parent educators and making a difference in the lives of more than 5,000 families. Several mothers reflected on their experience in the program, as follows.

> Realistically, the cost of groceries just makes it harder but with that they gave me ideas for how to afford it and still eat healthy . . . . I think one of them for me was for spaghetti dinners, not to add all the beef but add turkey, and I think she said for the noodles, wheat is better – not that I have to buy the expensive food, but little things like that.
>
> I think mostly for me it's just living where we live, it's so hot . . . what they helped me do is little work out videos, or even like simple stretches, or little yoga things for me and the babies to do together. It doesn't have to be so difficult or a whole preparation, but simple things you can do at home.
>
> [My parent educator] gave me little recipe books or when we would go to little events with Parents as Teachers, they would have examples of the snacks like I said, the little rice cake with cream cheese or the ants on a log. And it's just nice to have the ideas. Of course, every parent wants to do the healthy thing, but nobody knows where to start. And every parent, especially being a single mom, [wants] to do the easy route first and sometimes everything is five steps or six steps, so you need these many ingredients. And [this program] really simplified it; actually, broke it down, gave me alternatives. Instead of just saying, don't eat that, instead you guys gave me alternatives and ideas.
>
> [The program] made it more accessible to be able to eat healthy because everyone wants to eat healthy, but no one knows, like I said, where to start. No one has the information. For me, it was the first time as a first-time mom, getting all the information on how to do it and what's the right way to do it and here's some ideas and this is why. It was really, really helpful.
>
> Before I started the program, I thought that it would just help me be a little bit more consistent with what I was doing since I was already eating pretty good and things like that. I was thinking it would give me better options and just [help] me check in with myself and help me to become more fit as a lack of a better word. So, just continuing what I was doing, but maybe giving a little bit more tips. But because I felt derailed, then it was like I was starting at a level under where I initially thought I was going to. It did all those things just for me. It helped me way more than I thought I was going to need.

> I think it actually helps me, because like I said, even though I went into the program thinking this probably won't be that much of help to me, it came when I actually needed it. It was a really good reminder for me to make better choices, even as best as I could in the moment. I think it really helped.

Sleep During and After Pregnancy

Sleep is important during pregnancy and can affect an individual's physical and mental health, as well as relationships. In general, medical experts recommend that pregnant women get 8–10 hours of sleep per night.[53] Mild to moderate sleep problems (i.e., trouble falling or staying asleep, more frequent waking) are common during pregnancy due to hormonal changes, physical discomfort, changes in urination patterns, stress, and more.[54] Sleep disruption is also common during the postpartum period for similar reasons, and because of the need to take care of baby day and night. However, when sleep problems and/or deprivation become severe, this can lead to physical and mental health complications, as well as impaired caregiving.[55,56] To this end, it is important for providers to keep an eye out for warning signs and be prepared to make practical recommendations and referrals that will help pregnant and postpartum clients to get the rest they need. In some cases, behavioral therapy and/or medication can be helpful under the supervision of a healthcare provider.[57]

Employment Issues and Parental Leave

Several aspects of employment are important to consider during pregnancy and the postpartum period. On-the-job hazards such as chemical exposure, heavy lifting, and other risks can affect both maternal and infant health. On-the-job chemical exposure, in particular, has been linked to increased risk of spontaneous abortion, stillbirth, various birth defects, childhood health issues, and more.[58,59] It is therefore essential that those who are pregnant or thinking about becoming pregnant be advised about the risks of chemical exposure, particularly if they work in high-risk settings (i.e., manufacturing, laboratories, medical settings).

A different – but also critical – aspect of employment is maternity or parental leave. Leave is critically important for promoting physical and mental recovery from childbirth, and for parent–child bonding and family adjustment.[60] Research has also found that longer maternity leaves are associated with higher-quality parent–child interactions.[61] Leave guidelines and protections vary widely across countries, regions, and companies. For example, as of 2024, the United States has a federal law known as the Family and Medical Leave Act (FMLA) which provides up to 12 weeks of unpaid, job-protected leave per year for certain family and medical reasons, including the birth, adoption, or foster care of a child. FMLA applies to all public agencies, all public and private elementary and secondary schools, and companies with 50 or more employees. Additionally, many states and companies have additional laws and policies supporting paid maternity and parental leave.

Every parent and family deserves to take the time they need to heal, adjust, and bond with their new baby. However, as previously noted, not everyone is eligible depending on where they live and work, and many cannot afford to take unpaid time off of work. In the United States, low-income parents and parents of color are particularly likely to have difficulty taking parental leave.[62,63]

Putting It Into Practice

- ***Promote awareness of family leave options.*** Community and social service providers can be key sources of information and support for families regarding rights around parental leave. In the United States, this means being familiar with the FMLA. Examples of key facts to be aware of include the following.
    - All parents have the right to take FMLA leave, whether or not they were the one who gave birth (i.e., fathers, adoptive and foster parents).
    - FMLA provides up to 12 work weeks of unpaid leave in a 12-month period. These can be taken consecutively but can also be taken in separate blocks of time, totaling 12 weeks.
    - Group health benefits are maintained during this time.
    - Employees are entitled to return to their same or an equivalent job.
    - To be eligible, an employee must work for a covered employer; have worked 1,250 hours during the 12 months prior to the leave; and have worked for the employer for at least 12 months (months do not have to be consecutive).
- In the United States, it is also important to be aware of applicable state regulations and protections. Whereas FMLA provides job protection but not income, some states have passed legislation for paid parental leave. Paid parental leave typically provides a percentage of one's salary with a maximum weekly amount. Many other countries have paid national leave.
- ***Facilitate connections to resources and supports.*** Helping individuals become well-informed about the parental leave options available to them facilitates recovery, adjustment, and bonding with their baby. However, it should not be overlooked that in states without paid parental leave, it can be a significant hardship for many families to go without income for a period of time. You may be able to assist, especially with advance planning, by connecting families to supplemental resources. You can also brainstorm with them around resources they may be able to tap into through their support system. Unfortunately, this reality means that many parents must return to work sooner than is optimal for the health and well-being of themselves and their families. You can support them in navigating these challenging circumstances.
- ***Support self-advocacy.*** You can support parents' efforts to advocate for enhanced parental leave policies in their workplace and community (i.e., expanded access, longer leaves, paid leave). This might include helping them locate data that supports the benefits of parental leave for parents and babies, put together a proposal, and practice presenting the information.

Take Action

Take a few minutes to conduct an online search about parental leave policies in your local area. Who is entitled to leave and for how long? How can people apply to take leave? Knowing this information will help you to empower your pregnant and postpartum clients.

Intimate Partner Violence

Elena's Story ♥

Elena, a 32-year-old White woman, was pregnant with her second child. She and the baby's biological father had a tumultuous relationship that involved physical violence and emotional abuse. They broke up shortly after Elena found out that she was pregnant; however, he kept texting her threatening messages and showed up intoxicated at her doorstep on several occasions. Elena became afraid to leave her house and missed several prenatal appointments and outings with friends. When she did make it to the clinic, she did not feel comfortable opening up to the doctor, whom she had never met before. But with each day, she was growing more and more worried about her safety, and what might happen once the baby was born.

IPV is a serious, preventable public health problem that includes physical or sexual violence, emotional abuse, stalking, and more by a current or former partner or spouse. It affects millions of people, including at least 20% of women in the United States; racial/ethnic, socioeconomic, and other disparities have also been found.[64,65] Overall, it has been estimated that anywhere between 4% and 9% of individuals experience IPV during pregnancy and/or the postpartum period, with pregnant adolescents being especially vulnerable.[66,67,68]

IPV is associated with higher rates of reproductive coercion and lower rates of contraceptive use, which amplifies the effects of IPV on pregnancy and pregnancy outcomes.[69,70,71] Research has also found higher rates of reproductive coercion among individuals who are single, lower-income, Black, Latina, and/or multiracial.[69,72]

IPV can have a substantial impact on one's physical and mental health, including increased risk for physical health problems, depression, anxiety, post-traumatic stress disorder, and suicide.[73,74,75,76,77] It can also result in death. Tragically, in the United States, homicide is a leading cause of mortality during pregnancy.[78,79] IPV has also been linked to increased risk of adverse outcomes for babies such as preterm birth, low birthweight, small size for gestational age, and longer-term health challenges.[74,77,80]

Because of the devastating effects of IPV, the American College of Obstetricians and Gynecologists has been a strong advocate for universal IPV screenings before, during, and after pregnancy using validated, reliable measures. Despite this recommendation, rates of IPV screening remain low.[81,82,83] Research has also found that providing supportive interventions after someone screens positive for IPV can help to reduce rates of depression, decrease exposure to future IPV, and lead to better pregnancy outcomes.[84] Screenings and interventions are most likely to succeed when they are led by healthcare, community, or social service providers who are trustworthy, knowledgeable, trauma-informed, and culturally sensitive.[84,85,86,87]

Putting It Into Practice

- ***Take a trauma-informed approach.*** As a community or social service provider, it is important that you be aware of the prevalence of IPV and sensitive to the possibility that any of your clients – including ones who are pregnant or postpartum, fathers and other parents, and other members of the family – may have a past history or current experience of IPV. It is also important to be aware of your own biases and assumptions around this sensitive topic.

- ***Promote safety.*** When possible, conversations about sensitive topics like family planning or birth plans should initially happen individually with each partner, providing each person an opportunity to be heard and validated. You can then facilitate conversations between partners when appropriate to help ensure that needs are met for the most positive birthing experience possible.
- ***Talk with all clients about safe and healthy relationships.*** Your working relationship can offer a safe space for family members to share challenges and concerns, including those related to their intimate relationships. As this relates to IPV, you can do the following.
  - Provide a trusting environment.
  - Explore information and resources about safe and healthy relationships.
  - Support the individual in making choices related to their situation.
  - Facilitate safety planning.

Notably, experts have found that waiting to provide information about IPV until someone discloses that they are experiencing it may result in people not getting the support they need.[88] One option that addresses this is the Confidentiality, Universal Education + Empowerment, and Support (CUES) approach developed by Futures Without Violence.[89] This approach can be used with all clients and is designed to "[normalize] open and non-judgemental conversations about relationship quality and safety."[90]

Take Action

Does your organization use a standardized screening tool for IPV with all pregnant and postpartum clients, and guidelines for following up on positive screenings? If not, consider who you can consult with to put this into place.

Your Role as a Community or Social Service Provider

Listening and Learning

The data and information in this chapter present a picture of challenges to maintaining healthy lifestyles and relationships that families can experience during pregnancy and the postpartum period. Understanding the data, statistics, and stories specific to your community will help you to tailor your services to the issues, needs, and strengths of your local community and the families within it. Consider: what do you already know about nutritional challenges that those in your local community experience? What do you know about the prevalence of IPV in the community? What state-specific regulations does your state have for parental leave? How can you learn more about all of these issues (i.e., researching information and local data, listening to personal stories of different kinds of families in your community)?

Advocating

As discussed earlier in this book, your role as a community or service provider operates on two levels: (a) your individual work with families; and (b) your work with systems, including local mental healthcare. The lessons outlined in this chapter pertain to both levels of work and also point to the need for broader advocacy around a range of supports that help support healthy lifestyles and relationships during pregnancy and the postpartum period. You can advocate within your organization – for example, for coordination agreements with resources that make healthy food options accessible to the families you work with. You can also advocate within your organization for policies and benefits that go beyond the minimum necessary parental leave options. In addition, you can advocate outside of your organization in the community at large by lifting up policies, programs, and initiatives that support healthy lifestyles and relationships for all families.

Take Time to Reflect

Reflecting on the practice implications throughout this chapter and your role as a community or social service provider, what is one area where you believe you are already doing an excellent job? What is one area where you could improve your professional practice or deepen your knowledge and understanding?

Take Action

Now that you have reflected on an area where you could improve your professional practice, create a SMART goal to make it happen. Remember, a SMART goal is described as follows.

- **S**pecific
- **M**easurable
- **A**chievable
- **R**elevant
- **T**ime-Bound

For example, imagine that you have a pregnant client who is struggling to access nutritious foods. A SMART goal might be:

> My client Sarah is pregnant and having trouble getting the food that she needs. (**Relevant**). During our next visit (**Time-Bound**), I will give her a list of local food pantries and the phone number for the local WIC clinic (**Specific, Achievable**). I will follow-up with her the following week to see if she was able to connect with them (**Measurable**).

Key Takeaways From This Chapter

1. Nutrition, weight management, exercise, and sleep are all important components of a healthy lifestyle before, during, and after pregnancy which are also closely related to SDOH. Many people may benefit from education and support in these domains.

2. Work-related factors can affect both maternal and infant health and well-being. On-the-job hazards such as chemical exposure are major risk factors. Access to paid maternity or parental leave is protective, but also not accessible to many people in the United States and beyond.
3. IPV is a serious risk factor for negative physical and mental health outcomes. Universal screening is important for early identification and intervention.

References

1. American Medical Association (2023, June). *AMA adopts new policy clarifying role of BMI as a measure in medicine.* www.ama-assn.org/press-center/press-releases/ama-adopts-new-policy-clarifying-role-bmi-measure-medicine
2. Ayyala, M. S., Coughlin, J. W., Martin, L., Henderson, J., Ezekwe, N., Clark, J. M., Appel, L. J., & Bennett, W. L. (2020). Perspectives of pregnant and postpartum women and obstetric providers to promote healthy lifestyle in pregnancy and after delivery: A qualitative in-depth interview study. *BMC Women's Health, 20*(1), 1–9. https://doi.org/10.1186/s12905-020-0896-x
3. Zhang, J., Zhang, R., Chi, J., Li, Y., & Bai, W. (2023). Pre-pregnancy body mass index has greater influence on newborn weight and perinatal outcome than weight control during pregnancy in obese women. *Archives of Public Health, 81*(1), 5. https://doi.org/10.1186/s13690-023-01025-2
4. Diamond-Smith, N., Baer, R. J., & Jelliffe-Pawlowski, L. (2024). Impact of being underweight before pregnancy on preterm birth by race/ethnicity and insurance status in California: An analysis of birth records. *The Journal of Maternal-Fetal & Neonatal Medicine, 37*(1), 2321486. https://doi.org/10.1080/14767058.2024.2321486
5. Mendez, D. D., Thorpe, R. J., Amutah, N., Davis, E. M., Walker, R. E., Chapple-McGruder, T., & Bodnar, L. (2016). Neighborhood racial composition and poverty in association with pre-pregnancy weight and gestational weight gain. *SSM-Population Health, 2*, 692–699. https://doi.org/10.1016/j.ssmph.2016.09.008
6. Woolner, A. M., & Bhattacharya, S. (2015). Obesity and stillbirth. *Best Practice & Research Clinical Obstetrics & Gynaecology, 29*(3), 415–426. https://doi.org/10.1016/j.bpobgyn.2014.07.025
7. Mayo Clinic (n.d.). *Pregnancy weight gain: What's healthy?* www.mayoclinic.org/healthy-lifestyle/pregnancy-week-by-week/in-depth/pregnancy-weight-gain/art-20044360#:~:text=Amniotic%20fluid%3A%202%20pounds%20(about,about%202.7%20to%203.6%20kilograms)
8. Kim, L. P., Koleilat, M., & Whaley, S. E. (2016). A qualitative study to examine perceptions and barriers to appropriate gestational weight gain among participants in the special supplemental nutrition program for women infants and children program. *Journal of Pregnancy, 2016.* https://doi.org/10.1155/2016/4569742
9. The American College of Obstetricians and Gynecologists (2013). *Weight gain during pregnancy.* www.acog.org/clinical/clinical-guidance/committee-opinion/articles/2013/01/weight-gain-during-pregnancy
10. Goławski, K., Giermaziak, W., Ciebiera, M., & Wojtyła, C. (2023). Excessive gestational weight gain and pregnancy outcomes. *Journal of Clinical Medicine, 12*(9), 3211. https://doi.org/10.3390/jcm12093211
11. Yao, R., Park, B. Y., Foster, S. E., & Caughey, A. B. (2017). The association between gestational weight gain and risk of stillbirth: A population-based cohort study. *Annals of Epidemiology, 27*(10), 638–644. https://doi.org/10.1016/j.annepidem.2017.09.006
12. Monnet, A. M., Savoy, D., Préaubert, L., Hoffmann, P., & Bétry, C. (2022). In underweight women, insufficient gestational weight gain is associated with adverse obstetric outcomes. *Nutrients, 15*(1), 57. https://doi.org/10.3390/nu15010057
13. Fletcher, G. E., Teeters, L., Schlundt, D., Bonnet, K., & Heerman, W. J. (2018). Maternal conception of gestational weight gain among Latinas: A qualitative study. *Health Psychology, 37*(2), 132. https://doi.org/10.1037/hea0000555

14. Reid, A. E., Rosenthal, L., Earnshaw, V. A., Lewis, T. T., Lewis, J. B., Stasko, E. C., Tobin, J. N., & Ickovics, J. R. (2016). Discrimination and excessive weight gain during pregnancy among Black and Latina young women. *Social Science & Medicine*, *156*, 134–141. https://doi.org/10.1016/j.socscimed.2016.03.012
15. Champlin, S., Walker, L. O., & Mackert, M. (2016). Gestational weight gain through a health literacy lens: A scoping review. *The Journal of Perinatal Education*, *25*(4), 242–256. https://doi.org/10.1891/1058-1243.25.4.242
16. Kouba, I., Del Pozzo, J., Lesser, M. L., Shahani, D., Gulersen, M., Bracero, L. A., & Blitz, M. J. (2024). Socioeconomic and clinical factors associated with excessive gestational weight gain. *Archives of Gynecology and Obstetrics*, *309*(4), 1295–1303. https://doi.org/10.1007/s00404-023-07000-0
17. Makama, M., Awoke, M. A., Skouteris, H., Moran, L. J., & Lim, S. (2021). Barriers and facilitators to a healthy lifestyle in postpartum women: A systematic review of qualitative and quantitative studies in postpartum women and healthcare providers. *Obesity Reviews*, *22*(4), e13167. https://doi.org/10.1111/obr.13167
18. Hoover, E. A., & Louis, J. M. (2019). Optimizing health: Weight, exercise, and nutrition in pregnancy and beyond. *Obstetrics and Gynecology Clinics of North America*, *46*(3), 431–440. https://doi.org/10.1016/j.ogc.2019.04.003
19. The American College of Obstetricians and Gynecologists (2023). *Nutrition during pregnancy.* www.acog.org/womens-health/faqs/nutrition-during-pregnancy#:~:text=During%20the%20first%20trimester%20with,%2C%20yogurt%2C%20and%20fresh%20fruit
20. Harris, A., Chilukuri, N., West, M., Henderson, J., Lawson, S., Polk, S., Levine, D., & Bennett, W. L. (2016). Obesity-related dietary behaviors among racially and ethnically diverse pregnant and postpartum women. *Journal of Pregnancy*, *2016*. https://doi.org/10.1155/2016/9832167
21. Hromi-Fiedler, A., Chapman, D., Segura-Pérez, S., Damio, G., Clark, P., Martinez, J., & Pérez-Escamilla, R. (2016). Barriers and facilitators to improve fruit and vegetable intake among WIC-eligible pregnant Latinas: An application of the health action process approach framework. *Journal of Nutrition Education and Behavior*, *48*(7), 468–477. https://doi.org/10.1016/j.jneb.2016.04.398
22. Yee, L. M., McGuire, J. M., Taylor, S. M., Niznik, C. M., & Simon, M. A. (2016). Social and environmental barriers to nutrition therapy for diabetes management among underserved pregnant women: A qualitative analysis. *Journal of Nutrition Education and Behavior*, *48*(3), 170–180. https://doi.org/10.1016/j.jneb.2015.11.003
23. The American College of Obstetricians and Gynecologists (2024). *Exercise during pregnancy.* www.acog.org/womens-health/faqs/exercise-during-pregnancy#:~:text=Ideally%2C%20pregnant%20women%20should%20get,arms)%20in%20a%20rhythmic%20way
24. Arvizu, M., Minguez-Alarcon, L., Stuart, J. J., Mitsunami, M., Rosner, B., Rich-Edwards, J. W., & Chavarro, J. E. (2022). Physical activity before pregnancy and the risk of hypertensive disorders of pregnancy. *American Journal of Obstetrics & Gynecology MFM*, *4*(2), 100556. https://doi.org/10.1016/j.ajogmf.2021.100556
25. Watkins, V. Y., O'Donnell, C. M., Perez, M., Zhao, P., England, S., Carter, E. B., Kelly, J. C., Frolova, A., & Raghuraman, N. (2021). The impact of physical activity during pregnancy on labor and delivery. *American Journal of Obstetrics and Gynecology*, *225*(4), 437.e1–437.e8. https://doi.org/10.1016/j.ajog.2021.05.036
26. Sneed, D., Abeysekara, P. M., Slaughter-Acey, J. C., Giurgescu, C., Dailey, R., & Misra, D. P. (2022). Physical activity and its relationship with preterm birth in the presence of depressive symptomology. *Journal of Racial and Ethnic Health Disparities*, *9*(2), 670–678. https://doi.org/10.1007/s40615-021-00998-6
27. Zhang, J., Xiao, Y., Bai, S., Lin, S., Du, S., & Wang, Z. (2024). The association between exercise during pregnancy and the risk of preterm birth. *International Journal of Women's Health*, *16*, 219–228. https://doi.org/10.2147/IJWH.S447270
28. Yeo, S., & Kang, J. H. (2021). Low-intensity exercise and pregnancy outcomes: An examination in the Nurses' Health Study II. *Women's Health Reports*, *2*(1), 389–395. https://doi.org/10.1089/whr.2021.0011

29. The American College of Obstetricians and Gynecologists (2020). *Physical activity and exercise during pregnancy and the postpartum period*. www.acog.org/clinical/clinical-guidance/committee-opinion/articles/2020/04/physical-activity-and-exercise-during-pregnancy-and-the-postpartum-period
30. Lewis, B. A., Schuver, K., Dunsiger, S., Samson, L., Frayeh, A. L., Terrell, C. A., Ciccolo, J. T., Fischer, J., & Avery, M. D. (2021). Randomized trial examining the effect of exercise and wellness interventions on preventing postpartum depression and perceived stress. *BMC Pregnancy and Childbirth*, *21*(1), 785. https://doi.org/10.1186/s12884-021-04257-8
31. Kowalska, J. (2023). The level of stress and anxiety in pregnant women depending on social support and physical activity. *Journal of Clinical Medicine*, *12*(9), 3143. https://doi.org/10.3390/jcm12093143
32. Hicks, L. E., & Yeo, S. (2023). Longitudinal changes of depressive symptoms in sedentary women who exercised during pregnancy. *Women's Health Reports*, *4*(1), 523–530. https://doi.org/10.1089/whr.2023.0028
33. Forczek, W., Curylo, M., & Forczek, B. (2017). Physical activity assessment during gestation and its outcomes: A review. *Obstetrical & Gynecological Survey*, *72*(7), 425–444. https://doi.org/10.1097/OGX.0000000000000458
34. Rauff, E. L., & Downs, D. S. (2018). A prospective examination of physical activity predictors in normal and overweight/obese pregnant women. *Women's Health Issues*, *28*(6), 502–508. https://doi.org/101.16/j.whi.2018.09.003
35. Badon, S. E., Iturralde, E., Nkemere, L., Nance, N., & Avalos, L. A. (2021). Perceived barriers and motivators for physical activity in women with perinatal depression. *Journal of Physical Activity & Health*, *18*(7), 801–810. https://doi.org/10.1123/jpah.2020-0743
36. Kominiarek, M. A., Gay, F., & Peacock, N. (2015). Obesity in pregnancy: A qualitative approach to inform an intervention for patients and providers. *Maternal and Child Health Journal*, *19*(8), 1698–1712. https://doi.org/10.1007/s10995-015-1684-3
37. Lindsay, A. C., Machado, M. M. T., Wallington, S. F., & Greaney, M. L. (2019). Sociocultural and interpersonal influences on latina women's beliefs, attitudes, and experiences with gestational weight gain. *PLoS One*, *14*(7), e0219371. https://doi.org/10.1371/journal.pone.0219371
38. Anderson, C. K., Walch, T. J., Lindberg, S. M., Smith, A. M., Lindheim, S. R., & Whigham, L. D. (2015). Excess gestational weight gain in low-income overweight and obese women: A qualitative study. *Journal of Nutrition Education and Behavior*, *47*(5), 404–411. https://doi.org/10.1016/j.jneb.2015.05.011
39. Criss, S., Oken, E., Guthrie, L., & Hivert, M. F. (2016). A qualitative study of gestational weight gain goal setting. *BMC Pregnancy and Childbirth*, *16*(1), 1–8. https://doi.org/10.1186/s12884-016-1118-2
40. Kim, L. P., Koleilat, M., & Whaley, S. E. (2016). A qualitative study to examine perceptions and barriers to appropriate gestational weight gain among participants in the special supplemental nutrition program for women infants and children program. *Journal of Pregnancy*, *2016*. https://doi.org/10.1155/2016/4569742
41. Lindsay, A. C., Wallington, S. F., Greaney, M. L., Tavares Machado, M. M., & De Andrade, G. P. (2017). Patient–provider communication and counseling about gestational weight gain and physical activity: A qualitative study of the perceptions and experiences of Latinas pregnant with their first child. *International Journal of Environmental Research and Public Health*, *14*(11), 1412. https://doi.org/10.3390/ijerph14111412
42. Liu, J., Whitaker, K. M., Stella, M. Y., Chao, S. M., & Lu, M. C. (2016). Association of provider advice and pregnancy weight gain in a predominantly Hispanic population. *Women's Health Issues*, *26*(3), 321–328. https://doi.org/10.1016/j.whi.2016.01.004
43. Whitaker, K. M., Wilcox, S., Liu, J., Blair, S. N., & Pate, R. R. (2016). Provider advice and women's intentions to meet weight gain, physical activity, and nutrition guidelines during pregnancy. *Maternal and Child Health Journal*, *20*(11), 2309–2317. https://doi.org/10.1007/s10995-016-2054-5
44. Evins, C., Dennis, J., Mostert, K., Patel, S., Enyart, D., Eichelberger, K., Ewing, J., Tan, X., & Trilk, J. L. (2021). Exercise counseling in pregnancy: Do women perceive receiving the

information they need? *American Journal of Lifestyle Medicine*, *15*(4), 441–452. https://doi.org/10.1177/1559827621991851

45. Craemer, K. A., Sampene, E., Safdar, N., Antony, K. M., & Wautlet, C. K. (2019). Nutrition and exercise strategies to prevent excessive pregnancy weight gain: A meta-analysis. *AJP Reports*, *9*(1), e92. https://doi.org/10.1055/s-0039-1683377
46. Koleilat, M., Kim, L. P., Cortes, B., & Kodjebacheva, G. D. (2020). Perceived motivators, barriers and intervention strategies related to weight loss after childbirth among WIC participants in Southern California. *American Journal of Health Promotion*, *34*(3), 294–302. https://doi.org/10.1177/0890117119895948
47. Stang, J., & Huffman, L. G. (2016). Position of the academy of nutrition and dietetics: Obesity, reproduction, and pregnancy outcomes. *Journal of the Academy of Nutrition and Dietetics*, *116*(4), 677–691. https://doi.org/10.1016/j.jand.2016.01.008
48. Nagourney, E. M., Goodman, D., Lam, Y., Hurley, K. M., Henderson, J., & Surkan, P. J. (2019). Obese women's perceptions of weight gain during pregnancy: A theory-based analysis. *Public Health Nutrition*, *22*(12), 2228–2236. https://doi.org/10.1017/S1368980019000703
49. Haire-Joshu, D., Elliott, M. B., Caito, N. M., Hessler, K., Nanney, M. S., Hale, N., Boehmer, T. K., Kreuter, M., & Brownson, R. C. (2008). High 5 for Kids: The impact of a home visiting program on fruit and vegetable intake of parents and their preschool children. *Preventive Medicine*, *47*, 77–82. https://doi.org/10.1016/j.ypmed.2008.03.016
50. Cahill, A., Haire-Joshu, D., Cade, W. T., Stein, R., Woolfolk, C., Moley, K., Mathur, A., Schechtman K., & Klein, S. (2018). Weight control program and gestational weight gain in disadvantaged women with overweight or obesity: A randomized clinical trial. *Obesity*, *26*(3), 485–491. https://onlinelibrary.wiley.com/doi/pdf/10.1002/oby.22070
51. Haire-Joshu, D., Cahill, A. G., Stein, R. I., Todd Cade, W., Woolfolk, C. L., Moley, K., Mathur, A., Schwarz, C. D., Schechtman, K. B., & Klein, S. (2019). Randomized controlled trial of home-based lifestyle therapy on postpartum weight in underserved women with overweight or obesity. *Obesity*, *27*, 535–541. https://doi.org/10.1002/oby.22413
52. Haire-Joshu, D., Schwarz, C., Steger-May, K., Lapka, C., Schechtman, K., Brownson, R., & Tabak, R. (2018). A randomized trial of weight change in a national home visiting program. *American Journal of Preventative Medicine*, *54*(3), 341–351. https://doi.org/10.1016/j.amepre.2017.12.012
53. Cleveland Clinic (2024). *Pregnancy insomnia*. https://my.clevelandclinic.org/health/diseases/pregnancy-insomnia
54. Cleveland Clinic (2024). *Pregnancy insomnia*. https://my.clevelandclinic.org/health/diseases/pregnancy-insomnia
55. Jones, C. R. (2013). Diagnostic and management approach to common sleep disorders during pregnancy. Clinical Obstetrics and Gynecology, 56(2), 360–371. https://doi.org/10.1097/GRF.0b013e31828f2717
56. Lu, Q., Zhang, X., Wang, Y., Li, J., Xu, Y., Song, X., Su, S., Zhu, X., Vitiello, M. V., Shi, J., Bao, Y., & Lu, L. (2021). Sleep disturbances during pregnancy and adverse maternal and fetal outcomes: A systematic review and meta-analysis. *Sleep Medicine Reviews*, *58*, 101436. https://doi.org/10.1016/j.smrv.2021.101436
57. Wilkerson, A. K., & Uhde, T. W. (2018). Perinatal sleep problems: Causes, complications, and management. *Obstetrics and Gynecology Clinics*, *45*(3), 483–494. https://doi.org/10.1016/j.ogc.2018.04.003
58. Ford, A. R., & Scott, D. N. (2017). A critique of risk disclosure as the solution for minimizing toxic exposures in pregnancy: The case of nail salon workers. *New Solutions: A Journal of Environmental and Occupational Health Policy*, *27*(1), 51–67. https://doi.org/10.1177/1048291117697108v
59. Rahimi, R., Moeindarbary, S., Ghasempour, M., Galini Moghadam, T., Heydari, O., Ramazanian Bafghi, Z., Norouziasl, S., Abdi, F., Ashrafinia, F., & Dadshahi, S. (2020). Maternal occupational exposures and adverse pregnancy outcomes: An overview of meta-analysis. *International Journal of Pediatrics*, *8*(5), 11341–11346. https://doi.org/10.22038/ijp.2020.47228.3830
60. Irish, A. M., White, J. S., Modrek, S., & Hamad, R. (2021). Paid family leave and mental health in the U.S.: A quasi-experimental study of state policies. *American Journal of Preventive Medicine*, *61*(2), 182–191. https://doi.org/10.1016/j.amepre.2021.03.018

61. Plotka, R., & Busch-Rossnagel, N. A. (2018). The role of length of maternity leave in supporting mother-child interactions and attachment security among American mothers and their infants. *International Journal of Child Care and Education Policy*, *12*(2).
62. Goodman, J. M., Williams, C., & Dow, W. H. (2021). Racial/ethnic inequities in paid parental leave access. *Health Equity*, *5*(1), 738–749. https://doi.org/10.1089/heq.2021.0001
63. Elser, H., Williams, C., Dow, W. H., & Goodman, J. M. (2022). Inequities in paid parental leave across industry and occupational class: Drivers and simulated policy remedies. *SSM–Population Health*, *18*, 101045. https://doi.org/10.1016/j.ssmph.2022.101045
64. Cho, H. (2012). Racial differences in the prevalence of intimate partner violence against women and associated factors. *Journal of Interpersonal Violence*, *27*(2), 344–363. https://doi.org/10.1177/0886260511416469
65. Malcoe, L. H., Duran, B. M., & Montgomery, J. M. (2004). Socioeconomic disparities in intimate partner violence against Native American women: A cross-sectional study. *BMC Medicine*, *2*, 20. https://doi.org/10.1186/1741-7015-2-20
66. Bekaert, S., & SmithBattle, L. (2016). Teen mothers' experience of intimate partner violence. *Advances in Nursing Science*, *39*(3), 272–290. https://doi.org/10.1097/ANS.0000000000000129
67. Hahn, C. K., Gilmore, A. K., Aguayo, R. O., & Rheingold, A. A. (2018). Perinatal intimate partner violence. *Obstetrics and Gynecology Clinics of North America*, *45*(3), 535–547. https://doi.org/10.1016/j.ogc.2018.04.008
68. Kan, M. L., Palen, L. A., Hill, J., Herrman, J. W., Williams, J. D., & Feinberg, M. E. (2021). Preventing intimate partner violence among teen mothers: A pilot study. *Journal of Child and Family Studies*, *30*(1), 87–97. https://doi.org/10.1007/s10826-020-01831-0
69. Grace, K. T., & Anderson, J. C. (2018). Reproductive coercion: A systematic review. *Trauma, Violence, & Abuse*, *19*(4), 371–390. https://doi.org/10.1177/1524838016663935
70. Maxwell, L., Devries, K., Zionts, D., Alhusen, J. L., & Campbell, J. (2015). Estimating the effect of intimate partner violence on women's use of contraception: A systematic review and meta-analysis. *PLoS One*, *10*(2), e0118234. https://doi.org/10.1371/journal.pone.0118234
71. Rozario, S. S., Gondwe, T., & Masho, S. W. (2021). Pre-pregnancy intimate partner violence and short interbirth interval: The role of insurance status. *Journal of Interpersonal Violence*, *36*(23–24), 11260–11280. https://doi.org/10.1177/0886260519897325
72. Grace, K. T., Decker, M. R., Alexander, K. A., Campbell, J., Miller, E., Perrin, N., & Glass, N. (2022). Reproductive coercion, intimate partner violence, and unintended pregnancy among Latina women. *Journal of Interpersonal Violence*, *37*(3–4), 1604–1636. https://doi.org/10.1177/0886260520922363
73. Bonomi, A. E., Anderson, M. L., Rivara, F. P., & Thompson, R. S. (2007). Health outcomes in women with physical and sexual intimate partner violence exposure. *Journal of Women's Health (2002)*, *16*(7), 987–997. https://doi.org/10.1089/jwh.2006.0239
74. Al-Marhabi, B. D., Fahim, W. A., Katooa, N. E., & Al-Nujaydi, A. A. (2023). Maternal and fetal outcomes among pregnant women exposed to violence. *Cureus*, *15*(9), e44715. https://doi.org/10.7759/cureus.44715
75. Perez, G. R., Stasik-O'Brien, S. M., Laifer, L. M., & Brock, R. L. (2022). Psychological and physical intimate partner aggression are associated with broad and specific internalizing symptoms during pregnancy. *International Journal of Environmental Research and Public Health*, *19*(3), 1662. https://doi.org/10.3390/ijerph19031662
76. Goldstein, B. L., Briggs-Gowan, M., & Grasso, D. J. (2021). The effects of intimate partner violence and a history of childhood abuse on mental health and stress during pregnancy. *Journal of Family Violence*, *36*(3), 337–346. https://doi.org/10.1007/s10896-020-00149-1
77. Greely, J. T., Dongarwar, D., Crear, L., Adeyeye, M., Reyna-Carrillo, A., & Salihu, H. M. (2022). Violence against pregnant women and adverse maternal/fetal outcomes in the United States: Racial/ethnic disparities. *Women & Health*, *62*(6), 513–521. https://doi.org/10.1080/03630242.2022.2074610
78. Modest, A. M., Prater, L. C., & Joseph, N. T. (2022). Pregnancy-associated homicide and suicide: An analysis of the National Violent Death Reporting System, 2008–2019. *Obstetrics and Gynecology*, *140*(4), 565–573. https://doi.org/10.1097/AOG.0000000000004932
79. Morrison, P. K., Pallatino, C., Fusco, R. A., Kenkre, T., Chang, J., & Krans, E. E. (2022). Pregnant victims of intimate partner homicide in the national violent death reporting

system database, 2003–2014: A descriptive analysis. *Journal of Interpersonal Violence*, *37*(5–6), NP2652–NP2670. https://doi.org/10.1177/0886260520943726

80. Kim, J. Y., Zhang, L., Gruber, A. M., Kim, S. K., Holmes, M. R., & Brevda, A. (2024). Prenatal exposure to intimate partner violence and child developmental outcomes: A scoping review study. *Trauma, Violence & Abuse*, *25*(3), 2249–2263. https://doi.org/10.1177/15248380231209434
81. Chisholm, C. A., Bullock, L., & Ferguson, J. E. J., II (2017b). Intimate partner violence and pregnancy: Screening and intervention. *American Journal of Obstetrics and Gynecology*, *217*(2), 145–149. https://doi.org/10.1016/j.ajog.2017.05.043
82. Kozhimannil, K. B., Lewis, V. A., Interrante, J. D., Chastain, P. L., & Admon, L. (2023). Screening for and experiences of intimate partner violence in the United States before, during, and after pregnancy, 2016–2019. *American Journal of Public Health*, *113*(3), 297–305. https://doi.org/10.2105/AJPH.2022.307195
83. Travers, C. S., Devereux, P. G., & Yang, W. (2021). Prevalence and screening of intimate partner violence and association with neonatal low birth weight. *Journal of Family Violence*, *36*(4), 399–406. https://doi.org/10.1007/s10896-020-00203-y
84. Alhusen, J. L., Ray, E., Sharps, P., & Bullock, L. (2015). Intimate partner violence during pregnancy: Maternal and neonatal outcomes. *Journal of Women's Health*, *24*(1), 100–106. https://doi.org/10.1089/jwh.2014.4872
85. Muñoz, E. A., Le, V. D., Lu, Y., Shorey, R. C., & Temple, J. R. (2023). Reproductive coercion and intimate partner violence victimization among a racially and ethnically diverse young adult sample. *Journal of Interpersonal Violence*, *38*(1–2), NP1261–NP1278. https://doi.org/10.1177/08862605221092349
86. Schaefer, L. M., Howell, K. H., Sheddan, H. C., Napier, T. R., Shoemaker, H. L., & Miller-Graff, L. E. (2021). The road to resilience: Strength and coping among pregnant women exposed to intimate partner violence. *Journal of Interpersonal Violence*, *36*(17–18), 8382–8408. https://doi.org/10.1177/0886260519850538
87. Battaglia, T. A., Finley, E., & Liebschutz, J. M. (2003). Survivors of intimate partner violence speak out: Trust in the patient-provider relationship. *Journal of General Internal Medicine*, *18*(8), 617–623. https://doi.org/10.1046/j.1525-1497.2003.21013.x
88. Reproductive Health National Training Center (2022). *Moving beyond screening for IPV: Understanding the CUES intervention webinar.* https://rhntc.org/resources/moving-beyond-screening-ipv-understanding-cues-webinar
89. Miller, E. (2019). *The evidence behind CUES: An intervention to address intimate partner violence in health settings.* www.futureswithoutviolence.org/wp-content/uploads/CUES-Graphic-and-Evidence-2020.pdf
90. National Health Resource Center on Domestic Violence (n.d.). *Connected Parents, Connected Kids (CPCK).* https://store.futureswithoutviolence.org/wp-content/uploads/2020/06/CPCK_Infosheet-Final-Print_11.22-PDF.pdf

10 Synthesis and Call to Action

Former U.S. President Barack Obama has said: "Change will not come if we wait for some other person or some other time. We are the ones we've been waiting for. We are the change that we seek."[1]

While there are many reasons to be frustrated, despair, and feel helpless about the experiences of pregnant and postpartum families that we have described in this book, there are also many reasons to hope. One large reason for hope is the evolving role of community and social service providers like yourself to support families through pregnancy and beyond. There is growing consensus that medical professionals alone cannot solve the problem of maternal and infant morbidity and mortality. It requires a village – a truly cross-disciplinary, collaborative effort – to give families the support they need, and deserve, during this vulnerable and transformative time of life. You are a part of that village.

Most importantly, beyond the tangible education, resources, and interventions that you can offer, there is power in the trusting relationships that you build with families as they move through pregnancy and beyond. This is particularly true when working with families from backgrounds that have been historically marginalized or mistreated by the healthcare and social service systems, and who are at increased risk for health complications during and after pregnancy. The steady presence of a caring, capable community or social service provider like yourself can give families the safe space they need to open up about their experiences, seek and accept support, and have the confidence to advocate for themselves and their babies. These relationships are the very best hope for promoting healthy outcomes for pregnant and postpartum individuals, babies, and families. As the Reverend Jennifer Bailey has said, "Relationships move at the speed of trust, but social change moves at the speed of relationships."[2]

Around the world, far too many experience preventable health complications and even death during pregnancy, childbirth, and the first year after birth – despite the medical advancements of recent decades. Some groups – for example, people of color, those with low incomes, those who identify as LGTBQ+, and those with disabilities – are at particularly high risk for negative outcomes. These groups are at increased risk not because there is something inherently wrong with their bodies or behavior but rather because of disparities in SDOH and the role that bias may play in how healthcare professionals identify and respond to complications and concerns.

This is where you, along with other community and social service providers – home visitors, community health workers, health education specialists, social workers, doulas, therapists and counselors, parent educators, and the like – come in. Because you work with families in their homes and communities, you get to know a bigger picture of their experiences than their healthcare providers, who may only see them on a

DOI: 10.4324/9781003476474-10

limited basis in an office. By partnering with families, you can work together to address the impacts of the SDOH on their pregnancy and growing baby. Because of this, we strongly believe that your work can make a meaningful difference in their lives and health outcomes.

You may be worried or unsure about supporting families during pregnancy and the postpartum period because you do not want to overstep your professional bounds or delve into medical issues too deeply. These feelings are understandable, but with the right knowledge and support, you and the families you work with can gain a clearer understanding of what your role is and is not. Indeed, community and social service providers can support healthy pregnancy outcomes without providing medical advice outside the scope of your training. What *is* well within the scope of the training and job descriptions of many community and social service professionals includes the following.

- Educating yourself and others about health issues that affect maternal and infant health, and hearing stories from your community;
- Providing emotional support;
- Conducting basic screenings for basic needs (i.e., food, housing), social needs (i.e., domestic violence), substance use, and depression and anxiety, and facilitating connections to appropriate resources;
- Offering basic education about the physical and social/emotional changes that occur during pregnancy and the postpartum period;
- Offering basic education about taking care of an infant;
- Reinforcing the importance of regular healthcare during pregnancy, the postpartum period, and the first year of life, as well as providing referrals to trusted providers;
- Coaching pregnant and postpartum clients and their support systems around advocating for themselves;
- And more.

We hope that after reading this book, you feel affirmed in the importance of your role as we all work together to reduce the unacceptably high rate of health problems/complications and death during pregnancy and beyond. We leave you with some key recommendations for community and social service providers that were offered throughout this book. These tables remind you of key content to cover with pregnant and postpartum families, areas for professional development, continuous quality improvement at the organizational and/or systems levels, community collaborations and referral processes, and broader advocacy. Remember: you cannot and do not need to address all these factors at once or on your own. We encourage you to start by identifying one item in each category about which you feel most passionately or that you believe is a significant need for your community or organization.

As you review the suggestions in Tables 10.1–10.3, and the others throughout this book, we hope that you can see your role represented and also recognize how many other skills and roles are needed as a part of the solution. We encourage you to share your learnings from this book with your colleagues and others with whom you work, and to consider where you can lean in as you continue your very important work with pregnant and postpartum families.

Table 10.1 Key Content to Cover With Pregnant and Postpartum Families: Synthesized Recommendations for Community and Social Service Providers

Key Content to Cover with Pregnant and Postpartum Parents and Families
Consider whether you feel prepared to address the following topics with families, and whether you have related screening tools, informational material, or resources ready. Be sure that any family-facing resources are available in their preferred language and are written at an accessible level.
• Major personal and family health history (both physical and mental) • The importance of having a trusted social support system • Healthy relationships and IPV • Maintaining a healthy lifestyle (i.e., nutrition, exercise, sleep) • Finding a culturally sensitive healthcare provider and the importance of regular healthcare before, during, and after pregnancy • Family planning and contraception • Substance use during pregnancy and the postpartum period • Normal physical and social/emotional changes during pregnancy • Major topics and milestones around fetal development • Warning signs of potential physical health complications during pregnancy • Warning signs of potential mental health complications (i.e., depression, anxiety, and suicidality) during pregnancy • Creating a birth plan, including plans for social support during childbirth and the early postpartum period • Normal physical and social/emotional changes during the postpartum period and the transition to parenthood • Warning signs of potential postpartum physical health complications • Warning signs of potential postpartum mental health complications (i.e., depression, anxiety, and suicidality) • Safely caring for an infant (i.e., safe sleep, childproofing) • Infant feeding options • Legal protections for breastfeeding and pumping parents • Infant development milestones • Finding a pediatric healthcare provider and the importance of regular healthcare during the first year of life • Maternity and parental leave options

Table 10.2 Organizational and Systems-Level Supports and Improvements: Synthesized Recommendations for Community and Social Service Providers

Areas for Professional Development	*Organizational- and Systems-Level Continuous Quality Improvement*
Consider whether you or your colleagues/supervisees might benefit from additional professional development in the following areas, to increase your confidence in working with expecting families.	***Consider whether your organization has policies and procedures in place in the following areas, to ensure that high-quality support is being provided to expecting families, and to those of you who work with them.***
• All the topics listed in Table 10.1 • Issues related to cultural sensitivity and family values	• Timing, frequency, and content of visits/appointments during pregnancy and the postpartum period (including the days and weeks after giving birth).

(*Continued*)

Table 10.2 (Continued)

Areas for Professional Development	*Organizational- and Systems-Level Continuous Quality Improvement*
• Reflective listening, emotional support, and motivational interviewing skills• Administering and interpreting screening tools (i.e., for mental health, substance use, IPV) • Culturally mindful, trauma-informed approaches to sensitive conversations • Coaching strategies to support to pregnant and postpartum clients and families around self-advocacy, lifestyle changes, etc. • Raising sensitive topics and using supportive, non-stigmatizing language • Identifying and responding to a physical health crisis (i.e., first aid) • Identifying and responding to a mental health crisis (i.e., "mental health first aid") • Identifying and responding to a substance use crisis (including naloxone administration) • Identifying and responding to possible infant maltreatment • Supporting families experiencing grief or loss • Professional self-care	• Universal screening of pregnant and postpartum individuals in key areas (i.e., mental health, substance use, IPV) • Protocols for handling client physical health crises • Protocols for handling client mental health crises • Protocols for handling client substance use crises • Protocols for handling concerns about possible infant maltreatment • Navigating and providing guidance around potentially sensitive topics (i.e., contraception, pregnancy termination) • Continuing to support families which have experienced death during pregnancy, postpartum, or the first year of life

Table 10.3 Collaborations, Referrals, and Advocacy in the Broader Community: Synthesized Recommendations for Community and Social Service Providers

Community Collaborations and Referral Processes	*Broader Advocacy*
Consider whether you and/or your organization have strong collaborations and referral processes in place with the following types of organizations that serve pregnant and postpartum families.	***Consider whether you and or/your organization might be willing to donate your professional expertise to raising awareness and advocating around the following topics – locally, regionally, nationally, or beyond.***
• Basic resources and social services (i.e., food, housing, infant care items) • Trusted, culturally sensitive: • Medical/healthcare providers (i.e., obstetricians/gynecologists, midwives, nurse practitioners, physical therapists, nutritionists, pediatricians) • Mental healthcare providers (i.e., therapists or counselors, psychiatrists) • Substance use treatment providers • Doulas • Lactation consultants • Resources for those experiencing IPV • Childbirth education • Infant care education	• SDOH and access to basic resources and social services • Family planning, contraception, and related healthcare options • Maternal physical health complications and related deaths, including disparities • Maternal mental health complications and related deaths, including disparities • Maternal substance use and related deaths, including disparities • Access to high-quality, culturally sensitive, affordable healthcare (physical, mental, and substance use-related) during pregnancy and the postpartum period • Awareness of physical health complications and related deaths among infants, including disparities

(*Continued*)

Table 10.3 (Continued)

Community Collaborations and Referral Processes	*Broader Advocacy*
• Support groups for pregnant individuals, new parents, and families which have experienced pregnancy-related loss	• Access to high-quality, culturally sensitive, affordable healthcare for newborns and infants • Access to community and social services (i.e., home visiting, doula support, parent education) during pregnancy and the postpartum period • Rights of breastfeeding and pumping people in the workplace and community • Access to adequate paid maternity and parental leave

Key Takeaways From This Chapter

1. Health complications and death are far too prevalent during pregnancy, childbirth, and the year after giving birth. The solutions to this problem are unlikely to lie with healthcare providers and systems alone.
2. Community and social service providers can meaningfully affect pregnancy outcomes without providing medical advice outside the scope of their training.
3. The most promising agents of change are the trusting, long-term relationships that community and social service providers build with families during pregnancy and beyond.

References

Obama, B. (2008). Barack Obama's Feb. 5 speech [Speech transcript]. *The New York Times*. https://www.nytimes.com/2008/02/05/us/politics/05text-obama.html

Bailey, J., & Flowers, L. (2019). Cultivating brave space [Podcast transcript]. On Being with Krista Tippett. https://onbeing.org/programs/jennifer-bailey-and-lennon-flowers-an-invitation-to-brave-space/

Glossary

Atypical birthweight and/or size for gestational age: When a newborn is significantly smaller or bigger than expected based on when they were delivered (i.e., gestational age). Newborns who are smaller than expected are at increased risk for breathing, feeding, and temperature regulation difficulties, neurological and gastrointestinal problems, sudden infant death syndrome (SIDS), and more. Newborns who are larger than expected are at increased risk for injury during birth, breathing problems and low blood sugar shortly after birth, and more. Both conditions are also associated with increased risk of long-term health problems.

Body mass index (BMI): A commonly used measurement of the ratio of a person's height to weight, intended to serve as an estimate of relative body fat. In recent years, many medical experts have called BMI into question.

Breastfeeding: The act of feeding a baby with human milk, either at the breast or with pumped milk.

Cesarean section (or C-section, or Cesarean birth): The surgical delivery of a baby by making an incision in the abdomen and uterus.

Contraception (also known as birth control): The act of preventing pregnancy. This can be done by using a device (e.g., intrauterine device [IUD], contraceptive implant, diaphragm, condom), taking a medication (e.g., "the pill"), undergoing a procedure (i.e., tubal ligation), or through a behavior (e.g., abstaining from sexual intercourse altogether or during certain times of one's menstrual cycle with the intention of preventing pregnancy).

Doula: A non-medical professional who has been trained to provide support, education, and advocacy during pregnancy, childbirth and/or the postpartum period.

Elective induction: Labor induction that is initiated for non-medical reasons before the body goes into labor on its own (typically close to one's due date).

Family planning: According to the World Health Organization, "the ability of individuals and couples to anticipate and attain their desired number of children, and to plan for the spacing and timing of their births."[1]

Folic acid: Folic acid is a B vitamin that helps the body make healthy new cells. Everyone needs folic acid, but it is especially important for those who may get pregnant and who are pregnant. Getting enough folic acid before and during pregnancy can help to prevent birth defects of the brain and/or spine.

"40-day rule," also known as postpartum confinement: A traditional practice in many cultures that calls for a 40-day period of physical rest to allow the postpartum individual to heal, bond with their baby, and relax.

"Fourth trimester": The 12-week period after giving birth.

Gestational diabetes: A form of diabetes (high blood sugar disorder) that is diagnosed for the first time during pregnancy. Gestational diabetes is a serious condition which, when left untreated, can lead to serious health outcomes (i.e., hypertension and preeclampsia, preterm birth, need for C-section, breathing difficulties in the newborn, stillbirth) and even death. Like other types of diabetes, it affects how the body processes insulin. It causes high blood sugar that can affect both maternal and infant health. It typically resolves after the birth of the baby.

Gestational weight gain: The amount of weight gained over the course of the pregnancy. The recommended amount of weight to gain during pregnancy depends on several factors, such as pre-pregnancy weight, health conditions, whether there are multiple fetuses, and more.

Hypertension: High blood pressure. When left untreated, hypertension can lead to serious or even fatal outcomes such as preeclampsia, stroke, and placental abruption (separation of the placenta from the uterine wall).

Infant mortality rate (IMR): In the United States, the number of infants who die before their first birthday out of every 1,000 live births.

Infant mortality: Death of a baby occurring after birth, up until the first birthday.

Infant/child maltreatment: Abuse or neglect, including but not limited to physical, emotional, and sexual abuse; neglect and negligence; and exploitation.

Inter-pregnancy contraception: Contraception use between pregnancies to prevent unintended pregnancy.

Inter-pregnancy interval (IPI): The length of time between when one pregnancy ends and another begins, regardless of pregnancy outcomes.

Interprofessional care: A collaborative approach to healthcare in which professionals from different disciplines work together to provide comprehensive, coordinated, and patient-centered care.

Intimate partner violence (IPV): A pattern of physical and/or coercive behavior by someone who is, was, or wants to be in an intimate or dating relationship with someone. Examples include – but are not limited to – physical violence, emotional abuse, sexual assault, intimidation, and reproductive pressure.

Labor induction (or induction of labor): A procedure that uses drugs or other medical methods to start labor.

Lactation: The bodily process of producing human milk.

Maternity leave, paternity leave, or parental leave: A period of time during which parents are entitled to take off work to care for a newborn or adopted child without risk of losing their jobs. Policies vary widely across countries, regions, and companies regarding who is entitled to take parental leave and for how long.

Miscarriage: Loss of a fetus or baby relatively early in pregnancy. In the United States, losses are considered miscarriages if they occur at 20 weeks gestation or earlier. In other parts of the world, losses are considered miscarriages up to 28 weeks gestation.

Morbidity: Health problems or complications (physical or mental).

Mortality: Death.

Neonatal mortality: Death of an infant occurring up to 27 days after birth.

Out-of-hospital birth: Childbirth that occurs outside a hospital setting; for example, at home or at a community birth center.

Postnatal mortality: Death of an infant occurring between 28 and 364 days after birth.

Postpartum period: The 12-month (one-year) period after giving birth.

Preconception care: The medical care that a person receives in preparation for the possibility of getting pregnant.

Preeclampsia: A serious health condition during pregnancy or the postpartum period related to high blood pressure, which often involves bodily swelling and urination changes, among other symptoms. When left untreated, preeclampsia can lead to serious maternal and infant health outcomes (i.e., seizures, kidney or liver failure, blood clotting) and even death.

Prenatal period: The period of pregnancy (40 weeks if the pregnancy is carried to full term).

Preterm birth: When birth occurs before 37 weeks gestation. Preterm birth is associated with increased risk of health problems for the newborn, such as neurodevelopmental conditions, breathing and feeding difficulties, vision and hearing problems, and death.

Reproductive coercion: Coercive behavior in which one partner pressures, manipulates, tricks, interferes with, or threatens another into certain reproductive behavior (i.e., taking or not taking birth control, becoming pregnant, terminating a pregnancy).

Stillbirth: Loss of a fetus or baby late in pregnancy or at labor or delivery. In the United States, losses are considered stillbirths if they occur after 20 weeks gestation. In other parts of the world, losses are considered stillbirths if they occur after 28 weeks gestation.

Substance use disorder (SUD), or addiction: Per MIECHV, "A chronic and progressive disease characterized by an individual's inability to control their use of drugs or alcohol, despite negative effects and consequences."[2]

Substance misuse: Consumption of prescription drugs taken not as prescribed; drugs that are not intended for medical use, whether legal or not; tobacco; or problematic levels of alcohol.

Sudden infant death syndrome (SIDS): A sudden, unexpected infant death with no known causes, even after a full medical examination.

Sudden unexpected infant death (SUID): Any sudden, unexpected infant death. This category includes deaths from unknown causes, as well as deaths from known causes (i.e., accidents or injuries, including those related to how or where a baby sleeps.)

U.S. Institute of Medicine (IOM) recommendations: IOM recommendations are the guidelines provided by the U.S. Institute of Medicine (IOM). The recommendations provide defined clinical practice guidelines intended to optimize patient care and health outcomes.

Unattended birth (sometimes called "free birth"): Childbirth that occurs without a healthcare professional in attendance.

Unintended pregnancy: A pregnancy that is unplanned. This includes situations in which someone wanted to become pregnant someday but not at this specific time, and situations in which someone did not want to have any children (or more children).

Well-being: A state of physical and mental health, happiness, and good functioning in everyday life.

References

World Health Organization (n.d.). *Contraception*. www.who.int/health-topics/contraception#tab=tab_1

Maternal, Infant, and Early Childhood Home Visiting (MIECHV) (2023). *Understanding the substance use landscape*. https://cwlibrary.childwelfare.gov/discovery/delivery/01CWIG_INST:01CWIG/1222829740007651 . Accessed July 2025.

Index

Note: Page numbers in *italics* indicate a figure and page numbers in **bold** indicate a table on the corresponding page.